PSYCHONEPHROLOGY 1

Psychological Factors in Hemodialysis and Transplantation

PSYCHONEPHROLOGY 1

Psychological Factors in Hemodialysis and Transplantation

EDITED BY

NORMAN B. LEVY, M.D.

New York Medical College
Westchester County Medical Center
Valhalla, New York

PLENUM MEDICAL BOOK COMPANY
NEW YORK AND LONDON

Library of Congress Cataloging in Publication Data

International Conference on Psychological Factors in Hemodialysis and Transplantation, 1st, Downstate Medical Center, New York, 1978.
Psychonephrology 1.

Includes index.
1. Hemodialysis—Psychological aspects—Congresses. 2. Kidneys—Transplantation—
Psychological aspects—Congresses. 3. Renal insufficiency—Psychological aspects—
Congresses. I. Levy, Norman B. 1931-   II. Title. III. Title: Psychological factors
in hemodialysis and transplantation. [DNLM: 1. Hemodialysis—Psychology—Congresses. 2. Kidney—Transplantation—Congresses. W1 PS748F v. 1/WJ378 I59p]
RC901.7.H45I57 1978   616.6'1'0019   80-20681
ISBN 0-306-40586-5

© 1981 Plenum Publishing Corporation
227 West 17th Street, New York, N.Y. 10011

Plenum Medical Book Company is an imprint of
Plenum Publishing Corporation

Printed in the United States of America

To my children,
Karen, Susan, Joanne, and Bobby

Contributors

RAYMOND B. ANDERSON, M.Div. • Fellow, College of Chaplains, A.P.H.A.; Staff Chaplain, Department of Pastoral Care, New England Deaconess Hospital, Boston, Massachusetts

STEPHEN ARMSTRONG, PH.D. • Assistant Clinical Professor, Tufts University School of Medicine; Associate in Psychiatry, University of Massachusetts School of Medicine; and Adjunct Assistant Professor, University of Massachusetts School of Public Health, Springfield, Massachusetts

FRIEDRICH BALCK, M.A. • Psychologist, Psychosomatic Research Unit, University of Hamburg, Hamburg, German Federal Republic

SAMUEL H. BASCH, M.D. • Associate Clinical Professor of Psychiatry, The Mount Sinai School of Medicine, City University of New York, New York, New York

BRUCE H. BEARD, M.D. • Clinical Professor of Psychiatry, University of Texas Southwestern Medical School, Dallas, Texas

RICHARD BERNSTEIN, M.D. • Assistant Professor of Psychiatry, Departments of Psychiatry and Medicine, University of Vermont College of Medicine, Burlington, Vermont

FRED BROWN, PH.D. • Professor Emeritus of Psychiatry, The Mount Sinai School of Medicine, City University of New York, New York, New York

DENTON BUCHANAN, PH.D. • Director of Psychology, Royal Ottawa Regional Rehabilitation Center; and Associate Professor of Medicine, University of Ottawa, Ottawa, Canada

WENDY CANTOR, M.D. • Resident Physician in Psychiatry, New York University Medical Center, New York, New York

PIETRO CASTELNUOVA-TEDESCO, M.D. • James G. Blakemore Professor of Psychiatry, Vanderbilt University School of Medicine, Nashville, Tennessee

DENISE DEMAIO, R.N., M.A. • Pediatric Nephrology, Case Western Reserve Medical School and Rainbow Babies and Childrens Hospital, Cleveland, Ohio

ATARA KAPLAN DE-NOUR, M.D. • Associate Professor of Psychiatry, Hadassah Medical Center, Jerusalem, Israel

ALFRED DREES, PH.D. • First Resident, Department of Psychosomatics, University of Hannover, Hannover-Kleefeld, German Federal Republic

DENNIS DROTAR, PH.D. • Associate Professor in Pediatrics and Psychiatry, Case Western Reserve Medical School; and Rainbow Babies and Childrens Hospital, Cleveland, Ohio

HELLMUTH FREYBERGER, M.D. • Professor of Psychosomatics, University of Hannover Medical School, Hannover-Kleefeld, German Federal Republic

ELI A. FRIEDMAN, M.D. • Professor of Medicine; and Chief, Division of Renal Diseases, State University of New York, Downstate Medical Center, Brooklyn, New York

EUGENE B. GALLAGHER, PH.D. • Professor of Medical Sociology, Department of Behavioral Science, University of Kentucky College of Medicine, Lexington, Kentucky

MARY ANN GANOFSKY, A.C.S.W. • Staff Social Worker, Case Western Reserve Medical School; and Rainbow Babies and Childrens Hospital, Cleveland, Ohio

JEANNE HOPKINS, R.N. • Transplant Nurse Coordinator, Nashville Transplant Service, Vanderbilt Hospital, Nashville, Tennessee

KEITH JOHNSON, M.D. • Assistant Professor of Medicine, Division of Nephrology, Vanderbilt University School of Medicine; and Co-Director Nashville Transplant Program, Nashville, Tennessee

JORG KNIESS, M.A. • Psychologist, University of Hamburg, Hamburg, German Federal Republic

UWE KOCH, M.D., PH.D. • Professor, Faculty of Psychology, Department of Rehabilitation Psychology, University of Freiburg, Freiburg, German Federal Republic

MARTHA O. LEONARD, R.N., M.N. • Clinical Nursing Specialist, Rogosin Kidney Center; and Department of Surgical Nursing, The New York Hospital, New York, New York

NORMAN B. LEVY, M.D. • Former Professor of Psychiatry, State University of New York, Downstate Medical Center, Brooklyn, New York. Present affiliation: Director, Liaison Psychiatry Division, and Professor of Psychiatry, Medicine, and Surgery, New York Medical College, Valhalla, New York

F. PATRICK MCKEGNEY, M.D. • Professor of Psychiatry and Medicine, Departments of Psychiatry and Medicine, University of Vermont, College of Medicine, Burlington, Vermont

SUDESH MAKKER, M.D. • Associate Professor of Pediatrics, Case Western Reserve Medical School; and Rainbow Babies and Childrens Hospital, Cleveland, Ohio

ANDREAS RADVILA, M.D. • Former Fellow, Psychosomatic Medicine; and Clinical Instructor of Medicine, State University of New York, Downstate Medical Center, Brooklyn, New York. Present affiliation: Department of Medicine, University of Bern, Bern, Switzerland

FRANZ REICHSMAN, M.D. • Professor of Medicine, State University of New York, Downstate Medical Center, Brooklyn, New York

CARL RUNGE, M.D. • Associate Professor of Medicine, Departments of Psychiatry and Medicine, University of Vermont College of Medicine, Burlington, Vermont

TOM F. SAMPSON, M.S. • Clinical Psychologist, Southwestern Dialysis Center, Dallas, Texas

ROBERTA SIMMONS, PH.D. • Professor of Sociology and Psychiatry, University of Minnesota, Minneapolis, Minnesota

HUBERT SPEIDEL, M.D. • Department of Medical Psychology, University of Hamburg, Hamburg, German Federal Republic

JORGE STEINBERG, M.D. • Director, Psychiatric Residency Program; and Associate Professor of Clinical Psychiatry, State University of New York, Downstate Medical Center, Brooklyn, New York

JAMES S. STRAIN, M.D. • Director, Psychiatric Consultation–Liaison Service, Professor of Clinical Psychiatry, Mount Sinai Medical Center, City University of New York, New York, New York

PAUL E. TESCHAN, M.D. • Associate Professor of Medicine (Nephrology), Vanderbilt University School of Medicine, Nashville, Tennessee

JOSEPH G. TRAMO, M.S.S.S., A.C.S.W. • Chief Social Worker, Division of Medical Social Services, Temple University Hospital; Field Instructor, Temple University School of Social Administration, Philadelphia, Pennsylvania

MILTON VIEDERMAN, M.D. • Professor of Clinical Psychiatry, Cornell University Medical College; and Rogosin Kidney Center, New York Hospital, New York, New York

RAGON WILLMUTH, M.D. • Associate Professor of Psychiatry, Departments of Psychiatry and Medicine, University of Vermont College of Medicine, Burlington, Vermont

RICHARD M. ZANER, PH.D. • Easterwood Professor of Philosophy, Southern Methodist University, Dallas, Texas

Preface

Major nephrological and psychological organizations have, at best, set aside only small portions of their programs for papers or panels devoted to the psychological aspect of patients with end-stage renal disease. Thus, the increased need for information concerning the psychological aspects of end-stage renal disease has been met by occasional journal articles, professional peer discussions, small portions of national conferences, and informal conversations and consultations with people with clinical and research experience in these areas.

The First International Conference on Psychological Factors in Hemodialysis and Transplantation arose out of a need to have a forum in which the major people involved in treatment and research in this area could share their latest work among themselves and with the registrants. The initial encouragement for organizing such a conference came from the rank and file of nephrology social workers, nephrology nurses, and liaison psychiatrists and psychologists. In early 1977 I had decided that I would make an effort to organize such a meeting and asked the two other individuals most closely identified with major research in this area, Atara Kaplan De-Nour and Harry S. Abram, to join me in planning this conference. With their support and suggestions concerning the program, I embarked upon an attempt to raise financial backing for it. I was somewhat surprised to find that the many equipment and drug companies supporting nephrological conferences were not greatly interested in this one. Marketing considerations apparently play an important role in determining which conference they support. A conference headed by a psychiatrist does not necessarily result in tangible return in sales as compared to a conference headed by a nephrologist who will make continuing decisions in his clinical work for the purchase of nephrological equipment and medications.

Tom F. Sampson of Dallas who joined me as co-coordinator told me about the American Kidney Fund's work in financially supporting patients directly, usually when other sources are not available. He initiated contact with them on behalf of this conference. At a time in which no other organization would support us in a concerted way, the American Kidney Fund pledged adequate financial backing so that the program could be implemented. They also gave "scholarship" support to many social workers, enabling the travel expenses of many to be defrayed. The Department of Psychiatry at the Downstate Medical Center, under the Chairmanship of Dr. Robert Dickes and later Dr. Eugene B. Feigelson, accepted our request for underwriting some of the "red ink" which might have occurred if the registration of this conference was not substantial. Fortunately, this support never needed to be utilized. We are also indebted to the sponsorship of the International College of Psychosomatic Medicine of which Dr. Adam J. Krakowski serves as President and Professor Cairns Aitken as Chairman of its Educational Committee, as we are to Dr. Benjamin Burton of the National Institute of Arthritis, Metabolism and Digestive Diseases of NIH, the New York State Society of Nephrology, and the New York State Kidney Disease Institute, which also sponsored this conference.

This book consists of all but one of the papers presented at this conference, most of which have been updated to the time of publication of this volume. In addition, others were invited to contribute their work. These include the chapters by Drs. Drees and Gallagher as well as that by Chaplain Anderson. My work on this book took place during the period of time in which I served at the Downstate Medical Center as Associate Director of the Medical–Psychiatric Liaison Service and as Professor of Psychiatry.

The goal of this volume is not to review all the literature in this area or to completely cover the areas of psychological adaptation to hemodialysis and transplantation. All feasible sources were not tapped in creating this book. However, in publishing this book in which virtually all the major contributors in this area are represented, we are presenting the reader with a reasonable overview of what is known. As with my previous volume, *Living or Dying: Adaptation to Hemodialysis* (Charles C. Thomas, Publisher, 1974), I hope that this book will serve as an impetus for further research in these areas and as a guide for health care professionals in approaching patients with end-stage renal disease in a knowledgeable and empathetic manner.

I am indebted to others for their help in making this volume possible. I wish to thank Dr. William Mattern, President, and Mrs. E. Kay Hatch, National Executive Director, of the American Kidney Fund. I am also very thankful for the support given me by Dr. Eli A. Friedman, Mrs. Caroline Leto, Dr. Franz Reichsman, and Mrs. Marilyn Zwerin. Special thanks are also due Hilary Evans and Beth Kaufman of Plenum Publishing Corporation. Finally, I am grateful to my secretary, Mrs. Myrna Berger.

NORMAN B. LEVY, M.D.

Brooklyn, N.Y.

In Memoriam

The name Harry S. Abram was well known to me before I had met him in May, 1972. As a worker in the field of psychological factors in hemodialysis his name and that of Atara Kaplan De-Nour were the best known to me. It was inevitable that Harry and I should meet, and the occasion was a panel at the American Psychiatric Association in Dallas. I was confronted with an erudite, genteel scholar, a kind and humane man. Through the years, because of our mutual interest and growing friendship, we were in continuing contact with each other. About two years ago I asked him and Dr. Kaplan De-Nour to join with me in a three-person Steering Committee to organize a program for the First International Conference on Psychological Factors in Hemodialysis and Transplantation. As always, he was full of ideas aimed at making this a good conference. When I returned from a meeting of the International College of Psychosomatic Medicine in the middle of September of this past year, there was a sign on the bulletin board in the kitchen of my house saying, "Harry Abram died on September 3rd. Mary Lou called."

On that date, September 3, 1977, Harry Abram's death deprived many of us, including patients who have never heard his name, of an important person affecting our lives. His death at the age of 46 brought to an end the career of a distinguished psychiatrist, psychosomaticist, and psychoanalyst. Dr. Abram's childhood rheumatic fever and virtually asymptomatic rheumatic heart were important factors which caused him to focus his professional interest on psychological factors in physical illness. This is encompassed in an article published posthumously early this year in *The International Journal of Psychiatry in Medicine*. The scope of his professional interests included psychological aspects of limb amputation, pregnancy, the burn patient, heart surgery, obesity, hyaline membrane disease, and surgery in general. He was best known and internationally recognized for his early, continuing, and ground-breaking research on psychological factors in hemodialysis and in transplantation. He wrote prolifically about patient selection, was a senior investigator in the most definitive study on suicide among hemodialysis patients, investigated sexual dysfunctions of these patients, and described the major stresses of hemodialysis and transplant patients. Medical ethics and human relationships were an underlying interest in all his work.

Dr. Abram was a prolific reader and used his psychoanalytic knowledge in its application to literature in papers concerning Albert Camus, Joseph Conrad, Conan Doyle, Thomas Mann, and Stanley Weinbaum. He was a fountain of knowledge of what was current in many fields. A conversation with him, almost irrespective of the subject matter, almost always resulted in his relating the subject matter to a recent article or a new book in the field.

His soft-spoken, velvet, Virginia speech covered wide-ranging topics in depth and was casual and unobtrusive. Harry Abram was a gentle and learned man. He had a driven interest to give as much of himself as he could to his students, patients, colleagues, and family in the time he had available.

Harry Abram was a good friend, a loving husband and father, and a renowned professional. Those of us who knew him will remember his manner, his brightness, his kindness, and his wisdom. These qualities remain in our memories as well as in the other legacies he leaves: his family, and his many distinguished articles, chapters, and books. It will be a long time before there will be another person like him.

Recently there has been another death which I do want to mention—that of Samuel Chayette, a physician and the Director of the Rehabilitation Center at Emory University. He was a patient himself with end-stage renal disease due to diabetes. He was a leader in the area of the rehabilitation of these patients. Like Harry Abram, Sam Chayette was a mild-mannered, profound person with breadth and depth who will be missed by many people he knew, including the patients he cared for.

NORMAN B. LEVY, M.D.

Contents

I. Hemodialysis and Renal Transplantation

II. Hemodialysis

III. Renal Transplantation

I
Hemodialysis and Renal Transplantation

1

Uremia Therapy

Innovations Promise Near-Term Improvement

ELI A. FRIEDMAN

INTRODUCTION

Few universally fatal diseases have benefited from therapy to the extent that irreversible uremia has responded to maintenance hemodialysis and renal transplantation. Before 1960, when Scribner and co-workers devised a regimen for repetitive hemodialysis[1] every chronic uremic patient with the exception of monozygotic twin kidney recipients had no hope of living more than a few weeks once residual renal function fell below a creatinine clearance of 2 ml/min. In 1980, a choice of three effective therapies, each capable of prolonging useful life for years, are available to preempt death in renal failure (Figure 1).

UREMIA THERAPY LIMITED IN EFFICACY

Each of these regimens—renal transplantation, hemodialysis, and peritoneal dialysis—unfortunately has significant limitations and undesirable side effects. Transplant recipients lacking an identical twin must continuously receive cytotoxic drugs to retard graft rejection. These medications disfigure appearance, accelerate the incidence of malignancy, and predispose to bacterial and fungal infections. Peritoneal dialysis may be painful, extracts plasma proteins, and causes peritonitis. No peritoneally dialyzed patient is free from anemia or azotemia even though treated every other day. Maintenance hemodialysis, the most prevalent uremia therapy, also incompletely corrects the metabolic abnormalities of renal failure and at best allows patients to function less vigorously than if kidney function were normal. Because of these and

ELI A. FRIEDMAN, M.D. • Professor of Medicine, Chief, Division of Renal Diseases, State University of New York, Downstate Medical Center, Brooklyn, New York.

UREMIA TREATMENT 1980

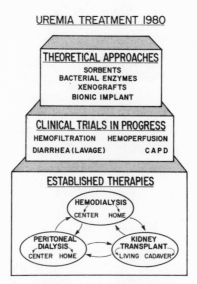

FIG. 1. Current therapies for uremia
are listed as the most promising inno-
vations which are in clinical trial or
theoretical exploration.

other deficiencies in current uremia therapy there is a quest for improvement in what are nevertheless life-saving treatments.

KIDNEY TRANSPLANTS DECLINING

In the United States there has been a steady decline in the proportion
of uremic patients treated by renal transplantation and home hemodialysis. The Greater New York region, for example, in 1978 was able to
provide transplanted kidneys for fewer than 200 patients who represented less than 7% of patients undergoing maintenance hemodialysis
(Figure 2). While media experts have promoted kidney transplants as an
essential and desirable component of American Society, the lack of improved cadaveric graft survival over the past eight years contrasts with a
continuously rising acceptance of dialytic therapy.[2] For the first years of
the 1980s it is probable that more than 9 out of 10 treated uremic patients
will be sustained by hemodialysis (Figure 3).

DIALYTIC REGIMEN

As currently administered, maintenance hemodialysis is a thrice
weekly therapy with each treatment lasting from 3 to 6 h. Assessment of

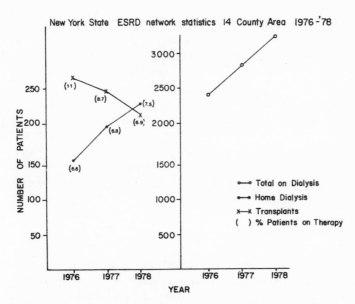

New York State ESRD network statistics 14 County Area 1976-'78

FIG. 2. Most recent prevalence data for New York region show a decline in renal transplantation despite a sustained growth in the number of patients on hemodialysis.

the adequacy of a specific patient's dialysis prescription is largely guesswork. Freedom from motor neuropathy, active secondary hyperparathyroidism, and debilitating anemia are necessary conditions to consider the clinical course of a dialysis patient acceptable. But, if health in its broader context is defined as well-being beyond the absence of disease,

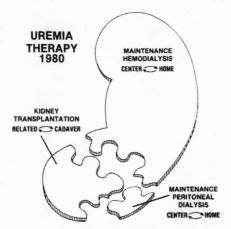

FIG. 3. An analysis of how renal failure will be managed in the early 1980s shows the strong dominance of hemodialysis.

then effective maintenance hemodialysis ought to permit active pursuit of physical and intellectual endeavors beyond marginal existence. Hemodialysis patients whose predialysis serum creatinine concentration falls below 10 mg/dl (a sign of sufficient dialysis) may nevertheless be unable to work full time, think creatively, or enjoy a normal libido. Schema for individualizing dialysis duration, blood flow rate, and dialysate composition according to one or another formula have not proven sufficiently clinically beneficial to allow for general application. Reliance on clearance or blood levels of marker molecules weighing 300–2000 daltons (middle molecules) for determining hours of dialysis is also of minimal value in predicting clinical benefit from a hemodialysis schedule. The technical aspects of hemodialysis have been relatively unimproved for 10 years. With the exception of recognition of the potential danger of a sustained elevation of parathyroid hormone blood concentrations, the renal fellow of a decade ago was equipped to function in a 1980 maintenance hemodialysis unit. Until more specific identification of uremic toxin had been effected, fabrication of different membranes for dialysis or alterations in dialysate composition are trial and error experiments with a poorly defined end point. Newer, smaller hemodialysis equipment, relying on the same principles of solute extractions as conventional systems are in clinical trial and will facilitate travel for the otherwise immobile patient (Figure 4).

CLINICAL TRIALS

Much excitement has followed the introduction of peritoneal dialysis without a machine. By surgically inserting a permanent plastic catheter in the abdominal cavity and exchanging a 2- to 3-liter fluid volume every 6 h patients can be free to travel or sleep while undergoing peritoneal dialysis.[3] Termed continuous ambulatory peritoneal dialysis (CAPD) this new approach to an old concept has won increasing patient and physician acceptance because of its simplicity and initially good results.[4] Speculation as to the proportion of new uremic patients who will be treated by CAPD have ranged from 5 to 50%. A relatively high rate of peritonitis is the current limiting factor to broader use of CAPD. For elderly, remotely situated, or unstable cardiac patients CAPD may very well be the therapy of choice even with its outstanding risk of peritonitis.

HEMOFILTRATION

Even the best hemodialysis or peritoneal dialysis-treated patients remain uremic (acidotic, azotemic, and anemic) throughout most of their interdialytic intervals. A majority of hemodialysis patients are hypertensive (blood pressure in excess of 140/90 mm Hg) predialysis. Alternative approaches to solute and water extraction, especially those that might improve blood pressure control are therefore highly attractive. Those experimental regimes now undergoing clinical evaluation are shown in Figure 5.

Hemofiltration, first terminal hemodiafiltration, is a technique in which solute and water are removed from blood under pressure across a semipermeable membrane with either previous dilution of blood (before it reaches the filter) or postfilter reexpansion of blood volume (after solute and water extraction). Hemofiltration is performed by combining blood hydrostatic pressure of 200–300 mm Hg and dialysate negative pressure to achieve a transmembrane pressure of 500 mm Hg, which results in production of an ultrafiltrate at the rate of 50–90 ml/min. Membranes employed have included polyacrylonitrile, polysulfone, and triacetate. At a blood flow rate of 200–300 ml/min, the amount of plasma water that can be safely removed from whole blood before increased viscosity and sheer forces cause hemolysis, protein denaturation, and/or membrane plugging is unknown. The plasma expanding fluid for either dilution or

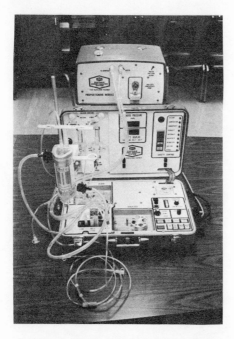

FIG. 4. A small portable suitcase hemodialysis system which will facilitate travel and dialysis in remote locations.

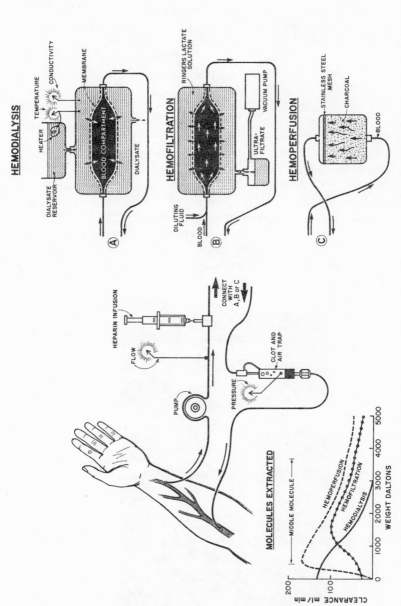

FIG. 5. The circuitry for hemodialysis, hemofiltration, and hemoperfusion is compared. Hemofiltration can also be performed with initial extraction of fluid from blood and subsequent reexpansion of plasma volume.

postfilter reexpansion contains lactate and magnesium and is otherwise similar to hemodialysate solutions. Patients have generally been treated thrice weekly for 4–5 h per treatment.

Comparisons of solute removal by hemodialysis and hemofiltration (Table 1) indicate that hemofiltration extracts a greater quantity of middle molecules (300–5000 daltons) than does hemodialysis. Proponents of hemofiltration as a sole uremia therapy cite better control of hypertension, reduced fatigue consequent to fluid extraction, and a higher hematocrit as its advantages over hemodialysis. Thus far, the technical complexity of hemofiltration has added additional cost to the equipment necessary to treat renal failure raising the per patient expense each year to more than $20,000.[2] Because of its cost and complexity the eventual place, if any, for hemofiltration is unclear. Until a well controlled A-B-A study substantiates benefits claimed for hemofiltration skepticism as to its superiority over hemodialysis is appropriate.

HEMOPERFUSION

Consequent to Yatzidis' report that exposure of blood from uremic patients to charcoal (a procedure called hemoperfusion) would extract creatinine and other nitrogenous solutes, this technique has intermittently been applied as a uremia therapy. Limiting the usefulness of charcoal hemoperfusion as a sole uremia treatment is its minimal sorbing affinity for urea and the absence of water removal from perfusing blood (Table 1). During hemoperfusion charcoal binds platelets and leukocytes to its surface, an undesired reaction which can be minimized without loss of nitrogen sorption by coating the charcoal with acetate or other polymers. Like hemofiltration, a major positive attribute of hemoperfusion

TABLE 1
Extracorporeal Fluid and Solute Extraction

	Hemodialysis	Hemofiltration	Sorbent[b] hemoperfusion
Fluid removal	Ultrafiltration	Ultrafiltration	None
Solute removal	Diffusion	Ultrafiltration	Sorption
C^a small molecules	High	Low	Variable
C^a MW 300-5000	Low	High	High
Current use	Uremia (sole Rx) drug overdose	Uremia (sole Rx)	Uremia (adjunct Rx) Drug overdose Hepatic failure

[a]C, Clearance.
[b]Activated charcoal.

over hemodialysis is an enhanced extraction of middle molecules. Whether combined with hemodialysis or hemofiltration, hemoperfusion is still very much an experimental therapy seeking a place amongst established alternatives.

INTESTINAL DIALYSIS

Daily secretions of nitrogenous substances into the bowel lumen are of a magnitude to attract attention to the gut as a possible substitute kidney. Every 24 h there are secreted into the bowel 71 g of urea, 2.9 g of creatinine, 2.5 g of uric acid, and 2 g of phosphorous. Extraction of a portion of these solutes from the bowel (which accumulate in uremia) has been attempted by intestinal gavage, induction of diarrhea, and feeding of oral sorbents.

Direct intraluminal perfusion of a portion of the bowel with a buffered dialysate has also been attempted. Surgical isolation and exteriorizing via double ileostomy of a loop of ileum whose blood supply has been maintained permits performance of intestinal dialysis. Uremic patients dialyzed periodically through an intestinal loop have biochemical and clinical improvement though severe renal failure (creatinine clearance below 2 ml/min) precludes the use of intestinal dialysis as a maintenance therapy because of inadequate solute extraction.

Other means of removing nitrogen-containing solutes from the bowel have been tried. Currently under study for this purpose are mixtures of oral sorbents containing charcoal, oxystarch (a urea binder), and locust bean gum which in concert could bind sufficient quantities of nitrogenous wastes to reduce or ideally to eliminate the need for hemodialysis or peritoneal dialysis (Figure 6).

THEORETICAL UREMIA THERAPIES

Other attractive ideas for substituting for missing renal function are in various states of bench or animal experimentation. The use of bacterial enzymes to recycle uremic wastes into usable metabolites is a rational objective. Why not, for example, convert urea in the bowel to an essential amino acid to rebuild protein? Cows can subsist on urea and sawdust as total nutrients because bacteria in their lumens convert these substances to protein precursors. Whether suitable bacteria can be host adapted to accomplish similar transformation in the human gut is unclear. Ingestion of capsules containing lyophilized bacterial enzymes is more easily

MULTIPLE SORBENTS FOR USE OF BOWEL AS A "KIDNEY"

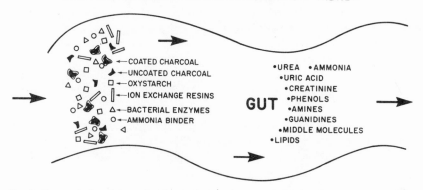

FIG. 6. Concept of a mixture of sorbents designed to trap multiple solutes are excreted in feces.

obtained though elusive goal. The concept of utilizing bacteria to recycle nitrogenous wastes is worthy of exploration.

Fabrication of a bionic kidney based on microprocessor control of miniturized implanted membranes and pump is an engineering assignment liable to solution. The technological problems have been largely solved. Implantation of a waste comsuming biological kidney substitute device which contains bacteria or specially adapted mammalian cells could combine microbiology with bionics. It is also probable that before the end of this century immunological barriers to the engrafting of kidneys from other species will be overcome. Should it be possible to transplant a bovine, porcine, or primate kidney without fear of rejection or intoxication, xenografting will supplant dialysis as the major therapy for uremia.[5,6]

SIGNIFICANCE

Irreversible renal failure has evolved from a uniformly fatal to a manageable illness with a favorable prognosis in the past 20 years. Current treatment strategies have deficiencies which reduce survival and limit rehabilitation. While renal transplantation and maintenance hemodialysis sustain tens of thousands in 1980, alternative treatments in clinical trial or still in a theoretical phase promise simplification and fewer complications. For the uremic patient treated today, the closing decades of the twentieth century promise benefits still only partially conceptualized. It is a safe bet that hemodialysis will, within a few years, be a therapy limited to historical medical texts.

REFERENCES

1. HEGSTROM, R. M., MURRAY, J. S., PENDRAS, J. P., et al. Hemodialysis in the treatment of chronic uremia. *Transactions of the American Society of Artificial Internal Organs*, 1961, 7, 136–149.
2. FRIEDMAN, E. A., DELANO, B. G., and BUTT, K. M. H. Pragmatic realities in uremia therapy. *New England Journal of Medicine*, 1978, *298*, 368–371.
3. POPOVICH, R. P., MONCRIEF, J. W., DECHERD, J. B., et al. The definition of a novel portable/wearable equilibrium peritoneal dialysis technique. *American Society of Artificial Internal Organs*, 1976, 5, 64.
4. OREOPOULOS, D. G. The coming of age of continuous ambulatory peritoneal dialysis (CAPD), *Dialysis and Transplantation*, 1979, 8, 460–461.
5. MANIS, T., and FRIEDMAN, E. A. Dialytic therapy for irreversible uremia (First of two parts). *New England Journal of Medicine*, 1979, 301, 1260–1265.
6. MANIS, T., and FRIEDMAN, E. A. Dialytic therapy for irreversible uremia (Second of two parts) *New England Journal of Medicine*, 1979, 301, 1321–1328.

2

Measurement of Neurobehavioral Responses to Renal Failure, Dialysis, and Transplantation

PAUL E. TESCHAN

The psychological factors to be considered in this chapter are likely to have two general orientations: (1) inward, toward *self*, and (2) outward, toward *interactions* with persons and things in the world—with components of thought and fantasy embracing both. There would be enough psychological factors for us to consider even if our patients were "simply" confronted with the coping stresses of a catastrophic illness. But in this presentation, your attention is invited to the fact that in patients with renal failure the problem is more complicated: the brain, the instrument of coping, of thought, fantasy, and interaction, is itself poisoned. And the treatment which relieves the poisoning itself creates both internal and external coping stresses at both physical and psychological levels.

Our general, integrating hypothesis is presented in Figure 1. In health, a normally functioning nervous system generates normal behavior. In many diseases the nervous system generates "illness behavior"—the more or less subtle behavioral changes which perceptive persons including physicians can observe. Sometimes such patients may verbalize complaints about self-perceived "unfitness," subjective symptoms if you will, as one feature of the generated illness behavior. This "generator" dysfunction also includes disabilities of another sort: Those deriving from impaired processing of incoming information into appropriate behavioral responses. Successful treatment restores health, which is expressed in normal integrated and interactive behavior.

The model in Figure 1 is easy to recognize in advancing renal failure. As renal disease reduces the capacity of the kidney to control the chemical environment of body cells—including the brain—the classic illness be-

PAUL E. TESCHAN, M.D., F.A.C.P. • Associate Professor of Medicine (Nephrology), Vanderbilt University School of Medicine, Nashville, Tennessee.

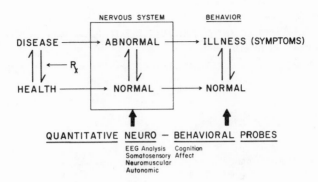

FIG. 1. Integrating hypothesis relating health, disease, nervous system function, and behavior and examined by quantitative neurobehavioral probes (see text).

havior of severe renal failure* produces progressive disability in our patients, e.g., sluggishness, lessened exercise tolerance, shortened attention span, drowsiness, insomnia, anorexia, restlessness, nausea and vomiting, a sense of coldness with hypothermia, myoclonic jerks, "restless legs," hiccoughs, asterixis, hypesthesia of feet and legs, torpor, coma, and convulsions.[1-3]

Some remarkable characteristics of these symptoms deserve our focussed attention:

1. They are generated by the nervous system, and may be classified as cognitive, neuromuscular, somatosensory, or autonomic impairments.
2. They represent integrated (illness) behavior in whole organisms.
3. They define and characterize the uremic syndrome clinically: they are the signals by which we identify the clinical uremic illness.
4. They disable patients.
5. They are rapidly reversed and readily controlled by dialysis, i.e., "merely" by correcting the abnormal composition of the body fluids; indeed they are among the indications for dialysis.
6. They are rapidly improved further (not always completely) by full restoration of kidney function, as by successful renal transplantation.
7. They are verbal descriptors, written in medical records to record observers' subjective impressions of the patients' clinical state.

---

*Possible synonyms: uremia; clinical uremia; uremic syndrome. However, these terms are often used to include some or all of the many other abnormalities (in biochemistry, cells, tissues, and organs) which occur in patients with renal failure. But in this presentation we use these words to connote the behavioral output which impairs patients' functioning in daily living.

We may note in passing the contrast between the neurobehavioral changes and the many other abnormalities in patients with renal failure. Those other, nonneurobehavioral abnormalities (1) are not usually symptomatic; (2) are detected at lower levels of biological organization[2]; (3) rarely disable patients; (4) are affected little or not at all by dialysis; and (5) recover slowly following successful renal transplantation.

Therefore, we have reason to be astonished when investigations of dialysis in "uremic" patients continue to ignore measureable neurobehavioral outcomes in favor of measures of these other abnormalities which are largely unresponsive to dialysis or irrelevant to the uremic *illness*.

When the uremic illness in patients is understood *as* a set of neurobehavioral phenomena it becomes reasonable to examine the generating nervous system function. Moreover, quantitative neurobehavioral probes instead of verbal descriptions (see Figure 1) are essential in the interests of objectivity, precision, and reliable comparisons between repeated observations. Accordingly, we have examined neurobehavioral function in normals, in patients with varying degrees of renal failure before beginning dialysis treatment, in patients dialyzed according to various schedules, and in patients following renal transplantation and during transitions between these situations.

The measurements included:

1. Power spectral analysis of the electroencephalogram to quantify the slowing of frequencies, i.e., the principal and common EEG alteration in renal failure. The power associated with the abnormally slow waves between 3 and 7 Hz was expressed as a percentage (EEG%P) of total power in the 3- to 13-Hz range.[4]
2. Maximum peak latency of the visually evoked EEG response (VER).[5]
3. Photic driving response: ratio of EEG power in the subharmonic to that in the fundamental (stimulus) frequency range; (PD S/F).[6]
4. Continuous memory test (CMT) of short-term word-recognition memory.[7]
5. Choice reaction time (CRT) required for decision between (visual) stimulus colors and a lever-pressing response.
6. Continuous performance test (CPT) of vigilance for detection of defined alphabetical sequences in a display series.[8]

The results may be summarized as follows for *all* of the measures examined:

1. The degree of neurobehavioral abnormality varied directly with the degree of renal failure.
2. The measures improved following onset of dialysis treatment.

3. They improved further following successful renal transplantation.

This *congruence* among and between the electrophysiologic (EEG, VER, PD) and psychometric (CMT, CRT, and CPT) measures is depicted in Figure 2. For each of the 6 measures the means of the data from our group of age-matched normals (N) without kidney failure is set at zero. The location of each group value for azotemic patients (A) not treated with dialysis (serum creatinine concentrations exceeded 10 mg/dl) is obtained by subtracting the mean value of the normals from the group mean of the A patients and dividing the difference ($\overline{\Delta x}$), for each measure, respectively, by the arithmetic mean of the standard errors $(\overline{SEM})$ of the N and the A groups: $SEM = (SEM_N + SEM_A)/2$. Similarly, the differences between the A group and that of the dialyzed patients (D) for each measure were factored by the respective $\overline{SEM}$, $(SEM_A + SEM_D)/2$, and plotted as shown. The process was repeated for the D $\rightarrow$ T (posttransplant patients) differences. Thus, three electrophysiologic measures (the resting EEG and two somatosensory-evoked potential measures) and three measures of integrated behavioral responses (involving short-term memory, reaction time, speed of decision making and vigilance) displayed similar variations in response to renal failure and its treatment. The objective data matched the expected comparative clinical state of these patient groups; and it appears that in renal failure at least, the brain's electrical and cognitive functions are related to each other: the "currents and juices" seem to be related to *thinking:* with obvious implications for the chemical changes of renal failure and dialysis on one hand and for psychological factors on the other.

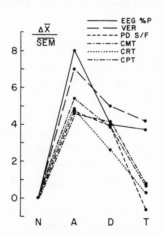

FIG. 2. Intergroup differences in means of each of six neuro-behavioral measures (see text).

It will be noted that the means of all of the measures achieve multiples between 4 and 8 times their average within-group standard errors in renal failure (N → A). Also, the EEG (%P) and VER which achieve the highest multiples (N → A) are on the average reduced to a lesser extent by the treatment, because differences between group means (not shown) are smaller and the average within-group variances are larger for these two measures in the treated groups.

Longitudinal studies employing repeated neurobehavioral measures over time in individual patients also reveal the same directional changes as the group data (see Figure 2) not infrequently at a subclinical level.[4] When similar data are aggregated to eliminate large and irrelevant inter-patient differences, the effects of transitions from A → D and D → T usually reach higher levels of statistical significance.

SUMMARY

In summary, neurobehavioral probes do indeed demonstrate variations in nervous system function which mirror the major clinical differences between normals and untreated and treated patients with renal failure. Subclinical responses are revealed. Subjective verbal descriptors are replaced by objective, numerical quantities. And these numbers are exquisitely relevant to the clinical uremic illness because they index at least some of its most characteristic clinical features.

Looking to the future, I recommend these further significant considerations to you.

1. Even if the endogenous, agitative–depressive uremic symptoms of renal failure have not progressed so as to disable patient entirely, his blunted cognitive and affective function may impair his receipt and processing of incoming stimuli and his orchestration of behavioral responses. We will need to remember at all times that we have a logical investment in optimized neurobehavioral function which dialysis and transplantation may achieve, since it underlies all of the adaptations and interactions which we will consider.

2. Hemodialysis as currently practiced, and even transplantation, improve but do not often normalize measurable neurobehavioral function. Comparable studies do not exist with respect to hemofiltration, or peritoneal dialysis, or to the treatment of blood, gut, and/or dialysate with sorbents. In our opinion such studies are both feasible and long overdue. Such further investigations of "uremia" and these treatments may now be released from their clogging bondage to conventional endpoint measures which do not respond to dialysis and only slowly to transplantation.

3. These quantiative indices may now make it possible to investigate

formally the causes and mechanisms of the uremic illness itself and of its response to dialysis, because measured chemical changes can be matched quantitatively to measured symptom-related neurobehavioral outcomes.

Finally, one can hardly overestimate the importance of trying to *understand* the dialysis-responsive, symptomatic uremic illness in terms of its causes and mechanisms. That understanding could just possibly transform the world of our present struggles into a world in which the original promise of our treatments may finally be realized, or at least a world in which patients may be afforded a more optimal neurobehavioral apparatus with which to confront a threatening illness and to achieve a measure of victory in their new life and living.

ACKNOWLEDGMENT. This work was supported in part by Contract #NIH-NIAMDD-2-2211, Artificial Kidney–Chronic Uremia Program, DHEW, and was accomplished by means of the collaborative efforts of Drs. H. Earl Ginn (Nephrology), J. R. Bourne and B. Hamel (Electrical and Biomedical Engineering), J. W. Ward (Neurophysiology, Electroencephalography), M. Musso and J. C. Nunnally (Psychometrics), W. Vaughn (Biostatistics), and by the technical and administrative assistance of F. Rogers, J. Folk, K. Streichert, A. Sanders, and several graduate students in biomedical engineering.

REFERENCES

1. SCHREINER, G. E. Mental and personality changes in the uremic syndrome. *Medical Annals of the District of Columbia*, 1959, *28*, 316–323.
2. TESCHAN, P. E. On the pathogenesis of uremia. *American Journal of Medicine*, 1970, *48*, 671–677.
3. TESCHAN, P. E., and GINN, H. E. In S. G. Massey and A. L. Seller (Eds.), *Clinical aspects of uremia and dialysis*. Springfield, Ill.: Charles C Thomas, 1976.
4. BOURNE, J. R., WARD, J. W., TESCHAN, P. E., MUSSO, M. F., JOHNSTON, J. B. JR., and GINN, H. E. Quantitative assessment of the electroencephalogram in renal disease. *Electroencephalography and Clinical Neurophysiology*, 1975, *39*, 377–388.
5. HAMEL, B., BOURNE, J. R., WARD, J. W., and TESCHAN, P. E. Visually evoked cortical potentials in renal failure: transient potentials. *Electroencephalography and Clinical Neurophysiology*, 1978, *44*, 606–616.
6. HAMEL, B., BOURNE, J. R., WARD, J. W. and TESCHAN, P. E. Transient and steady-state visually evoked cortical potentials in renal disease. *Electroencephalography and Clinical Neurophysiology*, 1976, *40*, 316.
7. GINN, H. E. Neurobehavioral and clinical responses to hemodialysis. *Proceedings, 10th and 11th Contractors Conferences*, AKP, NIAMDD, DHEW Pub. No. 77-1442, Jan. 17–19, 1977.
8. ROSVOLD, H. E., MIRSKY, A. F., SARASON, I., BRANSCOME, E. B. JR., and VECK, L. H. A continuous performance test of brain damage. *Journal of Consult Psychology*, 1956, *20*, 343–350.

3

Impediments to Psychological Care of the Chronic Renal Patient

JAMES J. STRAIN

INTRODUCTION

The end-stage renal patient is inevitably faced with multiple psychosocial problems evoked (or intensified) by his illness. Yet, by and large, he is deprived of the services which would enable him to cope with these difficulties. My purpose in this chapter, is (1) to discuss the nature of the variables that impeded the provision of psychological services to these chronically ill patients; (2) to describe in general terms the nature of their "psychological difficulties"; and, finally, (3) to propose a solution which would make adequate psychological care available to this population. The solution consists of a description of the psychosocial teaching program currently in operation at Montefiore Hospital and Medical Center, and of the mechanisms for funding which have made this teaching program a reality.

Although the psychological problems that confront the hemodialysis patient and their treatment have been discussed at length in the literature,[2-11] the nature and origin of these problems has not been specified in sufficient detail. Nor have articles been published in the literature to date that describe training or funding mechanisms that would enable the incorporation of psychological services as routine medical services in the ambulatory renal satellite setting.

JAMES J. STRAIN, M.D. • Director, Psychiatric Consultation-Liaison Service, and Professor of Clinical Psychiatry, Mount Sinai Medical Center, City University of New York, New York, New York. This work was supported in part by Alcohol, Drug Abuse, and Mental Health, Administration special training grant MH-13041 from the National Institute of Mental Health. This paper is an expanded version of: The liaison teaching unit: a funding mechanism for the psychological care of the Chronic Renal Patient.[1]

Impediments to Psychological Care for Renal Patients

Inadequate psychological care for patients with chronic renal disease can, in our opinion, be ascribed to four variables:

1. The structure and organization of the technologically-oriented medical facility
2. A lack of sufficient psychological knowledge and skill on the part of the nephrologist and the staff
3. A similar lack of psycho–social–biological knowledge on the part of the psychiatrist
4. The attitude of the renal patient toward psychological care

THE STRUCTURE AND ORGANIZATION OF THE RENAL DIALYSIS SATELLITE UNIT

In contrast to the acute in-patient hospital ward, the attending physician assigned to a technological clinic does not rotate; he is usually permanently assigned to that unit. Nor do patients rotate from service to service, clinic to clinic, or doctor to doctor. However, despite his extended "tour of duty," and the long-term "availability" of his patient, the attending physician has only a minimal involvement in the patient's treatment—on both a psychological and physiological level. Rather, delivery of the patient's day-to-day physiological treatment necessarily falls to the domain of the technician, and ironically the delivery of the day-to-day emotional support (in the treatment setting) these patients require also falls—by default—into the domain of the technician. The ascendency of the technician to the position of primary caretaker can be ascribed to four factors: There is a tendency, noted above, for the attending physician to be less involved with the direct delivery of psychological and physiological care. The nurse has become a "unit manager," and this move upward to administration makes her less available for her traditional function, i.e., direct patient care. Nor does the social worker necessarily provide continuity of care. All too often, he or she may be restricted to performing concrete services on behalf of these patients; the provision of ongoing emotional support is frequently viewed as lying outside his or her bailiwick. As a consequence of these alterations in the traditional roles of the nurse and doctor, and the relegation of the social worker to a more traditional role, the technician is likely to have more contact with the patient than any other member of the health care team.

THE NEPHROLOGIST'S LACK OF PSYCHOLOGICAL KNOWLEDGE AND SKILLS

The nephrologist's concern centers, understandably, on maintaining physiological homeostasis and the preservation of life. By and large, he has not been trained to manage the psychological problems of these patients. The psychological problems of renal patients may be particularly complex in that they are compounded by other issues: Competent psychological care of this patient population would require knowledge on the part of the nephrologist of the mechanisms of depression, pain, hypochondriasis, noncompliance, the organic mental syndromes, aging, and the patient's intrafamilial environment. In addition, adequate management of these patients requires a comprehensive knowledge of the effects of psychopharmacological agents. The staff, with the possible exception of the social worker, suffers from the same deficits. Ironically, even the technician who is most involved with the patient, and who theoretically might be in the best position to fulfill the patient's psychological needs, is most deprived of the training which would enable him to do so.

THE PSYCHIATRIST'S LACK OF PSYCHO–SOCIAL–BIOLOGICAL KNOWLEDGE

The psychiatrist trained in a traditional psychiatric residency may not be any more able—or inclined—to treat the psychological needs of these patients than the nephrologist. Typically, the focus of the psychiatrist's training is on the diagnosis and treatment of discrete psychiatric disabilities and functional disorders. But, apart from such considerations, the psychiatrist's attempts to deal effectively with the renal patient may be undermined by certain specific features of this disease: He is not prepared to deal with the patient whose somatic preoccupations and fantasies are not neurotically constituted, who, in reality, has kidneys that do not work and who is therefore machine-dependent for survival, or the kidney transplant patient who is dependent for his survival on one kidney which actually belongs to someone else. The fact that these patients have undergone a kidney transplant (from a cadaver, or a close relative, or a member of the opposite sex) means that they have, in reality, been penetrated, attacked, and surgically altered, that in reality they have incorporated someone else's body part. To cite another example, although the psychiatrist is trained to detect the presence of an organic brain syndrome, he may not be prepared to deal with a patient whose sensorium alters from day to day, secondary to diurnal oscillation in his physiologic status.[12]

Finally, the psychiatrist's competence vis-à-vis this population may be further diminished by his lack of knowledge not only with regard to the effects on behavior of drugs administered for medical purposes, but also by his lack of knowledge of widely used psychotropic drugs.[13] The point is that the psychiatrist, by and large, is not prepared to work in this setting. For example, with regard to the minor tranquilizers which are frequently administered to this patient group, psychiatrists are not always aware of the important fact that Valium is fully metabolized non-renally, whereas Librium is primarily excreted via the kidney

THE ATTITUDE OF THE RENAL PATIENT TOWARD PSYCHOLOGICAL CARE

The apparent indifference of the nephrologist and his staff, and of the psychiatrist to the psychological morbidity of the renal patient population is legitimatized by the patient's own assessment of his maladaptive behavior. Typically, he does not view his behavior as indicative of the presence of psychiatric disability. Rather, he thinks of himself as being understandably upset, anxious, disturbed, etc., and balks at a psychiatric label. In fact, there is some justification for this feeling. The concerns which beset the renal patient are very real: Will I be able to work again? Will my kidney shut down? What would happen to me in an emergency if my doctor is not available? Regardless of the patient's premorbid emotional status, stresses of this nature and magnitude would be expected to evoke some maladaptive responses.

Moreover, his reluctance to enlist the services of a psychiatrist outside the satellite setting is strengthened by practical considerations. Often, the patient with chronic renal disease must spend three days a week on the dialysis machine, which may compromise his ability to report for work (if he can work) on those days, with the result that he may suffer considerable financial hardship. Obviously, it would be unrealistic to expect him to visit a psychiatrist's office or clinic a fourth time within a single week.

SOLUTION

The four impediments listed above to the provision of psychological care for the renal patient are perpetuated by: (1) the persistent use of the standard psychiatric consultation model, rather than the liaison model; and (2) the lack of funding which would permit the establishment of a liaison model, and thereby enable psychological training for members of the renal team. The solution I propose to this problem consists then in the establishment of a liaison program, and in the creation of a financial base for such a program.

THE LIAISON PSYCHIATRY MODEL

Liaison versus Consultation

1. In contrast to the psychiatric consultant, whose primary function is to alleviate acute psychiatric symptomatology in the individual patient, the liaison psychiatrist focuses on all medical patients who are vulnerable to psychological disturbance by anticipating and preventing the development of psychological symptoms (primary prevention); by treating such symptoms after they have developed (secondary prevention); and by rehabilitating patients who have manifested such symptoms, in order to prevent their recurrence (tertiary prevention).[14]

2. The liaison psychiatrist participates in case detection, rather than awaiting referral; he clarifies the status of the caretaker, rather than focusing primarily on the patient; and he enlists the caretaker's alliance in the psychological diagnosis and management of the patient. In contrast, once the medical staff has identified the patient in need of a psychiatric consultation and initiated the request for consultation, it gains license to abdicate responsibility for understanding and managing the psychosocial needs of their patient. In short, the psychiatric consultant deals with psychiatric crises in particular patients, while the liaison psychiatrist attempts to gain a commitment from the medical caretakers to the effect that they will participate in teaching exercises which will enable them, in time, to take over much of the psychological care of the medically ill.

3. In essence, then, the psychiatric consultant remains outside the medical community. He makes only a limited attempt to disseminate psychological knowledge to other specialists; nor does he attempt to influence patterns of patient care. In contrast, the liaison psychiatrist contracts to become part of the medical community, and attempts to foster structural changes in the organization and operation of the patient care system.

Thus, within the framework of our model of liaison psychiatry, in addition to the dissemination of psychiatric knowledge and skills, the liaison psychiatrist is expected to be conversant with and conduct research in psychobiological mechanisms, pedagogic techniques, and group process; and, finally, if he is to achieve credibility, he must develop evaluation techniques which can assess the effectiveness of liaison teaching and intervention.

A Model of Psychological Medicine

Our model of liaison psychiatry must also be distinguished from earlier—and ongoing—efforts to disseminate the principles of psychological medicine, with respect to the content taught. Specifically, we have attempted to formulate a psychology of the medically ill which seeks to move beyond the descriptive model, which explains behavior in such terms as "stages of death and dying," "typical sequences of defensive patterns," and "the uniformity of the reaction of certain character styles to all illness."[15] Although these descriptions remain useful teaching tools, we believe that a more comprehensive psychodynamic adaptational model of behavior, and in particular, the formulation of developmental stresses and conflicts, affords an opportunity to bring a dynamic approach and schema to the understanding and management of the spectrum of psychological reactions manifested by the patient with end-stage renal disease. Within this conceptual framework, we have been able to evaluate not only the patient's reaction to the stresses evoked by this experience, but also the reactions evoked in the staff who cares for the patient, and finally, the dynamics of the staff–patient relationship itself. However, we recognize that, with regard to the renal patient population in particular, the content of liaison teaching cannot be limited to the psychological sector per se. For this group, he must develop and refine the psychological consequences of physical dysfunction on the one hand, and the physical consequence of psychological stress on the other. Because it has been our experience that the medical staff finds the psychological content of liaison teaching is most difficult to assimilate, this discussion will focus on this sector.

Our model is based on the premise that the caretakers in a renal dialysis satellite unit need to be knowledgeable with respect to the four intrapsychic parameters of psychological adaptation to chronic illness: (1) the patient's response to the psychological stress that is universally evoked by chronic renal disease; (2) the extent to which he regresses as a consequence of his illness; (3) the conflicts revived by this regression; and (4) the quality of the patient's current object relationships (and, in particular, the staff–patient relationship).

Psychological Stresses

Strain and Grossman have postulated that all acutely ill, hospitalized patients are vulnerable to eight categories of psychological stress.[15] These stresses are present in chronically ill ambulatory patients as well.

The Basic Threat to Self-Esteem and Sense of Intactness (Narcissistic Integrity)

Sudden illness, hospitalization, and the threat of death challenges the individual's belief that he is indestructible, that he is the master of his destiny.

If the disease has a successful outcome, this stress will diminish once the patient has been discharged from the hospital. However, it persists in the chronically ill, and in particular, when the patient suffers from serious chronic illness such as renal failure, which requires frequent treatment in the ambulatory setting.

Fear of Strangers

When the patient enters the hospital, he feels that he has put his life into the hands of a group of strangers to whom he has no close personal ties, and who may or may not be competent to assume responsibility for his survival.

When the renal patient reports to the satellite unit for treatment, he too feels his life is in the hands of a group of strangers who may or may not be competent to insure his survival.

Separation Anxiety

The hospitalized patient experiences anxiety because he is separated from important persons and things.

Because of the frequency with which the renal patient visits the dialysis unit, ideally one would expect that environment to provide him with the support and gratification necessary for his effective functioning. Unfortunately, too often he does not receive the psychological help he needs from the staff. Moreover, the fact that he sees patients who are as sick as he and dying is an additional reminder of his own mortality.

Fear of Loss of Love and Approval

This stress may be prominent, for example, in the patient who has undergone a mutilating surgical procedure. The renal patient fears the loss of love and approval because he suffers from a debilitating illness, is unable to return to work, or he may fear that his passive dependence on others will incur the disapproval of his family and friends, and the loss of their esteem.

Fear of the Loss of Control of Developmentally Achieved Functions

Severe illness may temporarily undo previously mastered physical and mental functions. Some patients agonize over the transient loss of these functions, and remain convinced, despite assurances to the contrary, that they will never be regained. For the renal patient, this fear has become a reality.

Fear of Loss of or Injury to Body Parts

Once the patient enters the hospital, his body becomes the property of his physicians, to do with what they will. His bodily fluids are drained; he is exposed, probed, and weakened. These hospital procedures require the patient to assume a passive–submissive stance vis-à-vis the physician, which may stir up frightening sexual and aggressive fantasies. The renal patient is routinely exposed to such procedures.

Guilt and Fear of Retaliation

Feelings of guilt and shame which may be revived by physical illness, and the patient's fantasy that illness and hospitalization are punishment for previous "sins" of omission or commission are a major source of psychological stress. These feelings and fantasies are prominent in chronic and end-stage renal patients as well.

Fear of Pain

Regardless of whether the patient suffers from an acute or chronic illness, the fear of pain cuts across all of the stresses listed above. In the vulnerable patient, each of these stresses may compound the basic painful experience, and, conversely, severe pain may increase the magnitude of each of these stresses.

These stresses are compounded in the renal patient simply by the fact that they persist in the ambulatory setting. For example, the acutely ill, hospitalized patient often is able to master the threat these fears pose to his self-esteem in the hospital setting by the use of denial or fantasy. That is, he may deny the severity, or even the existence of his illness. Or, there may be a reduction of stress once the acute stage has passed, and the feelings of guilt and shame that are typically reactivated at the onset of physical illness diminish in intensity.

However, once the patient is discharged from the hospital and must reenter the community, his capacities are actually put to the test. Now he must demonstrate his ability to perform successfully at work and sex, and to maintain satisfactory interpersonal relationships. Once he is confronted with the reality that his performance in one, or all, of these spheres may be impaired, the defenses (i.e., the use of fantasy and denial) that served him well while he was hospitalized may no longer be adequate. In fact, they may impede his adaptation. To illustrate, for the ambulatory patient who denies, or, more accurately, is unable to accept his limitations, the sheer effort of maintaining a facade of well-being in the face of actual physical disability will, in itself, constitute a chronic stress. And this is particularly true of the patient whose self-esteem is contingent upon his performance, which he believes is essential to retaining the love and approval of others.

Regression

Illness, which necessitates the curtailment of activity, and submission to medical caretakers and procedures, sets in motion the psychological regression that is an innate property of mental life. The ability to follow orders, to let others "take over"—in short, to adopt a dependent life style—is usually essential to the patient's survival during the acute stage of his illness. It may also be necessary throughout a chronic illness, such as renal disease. The point is that regression is not pathological per se; it becomes pathological only when the patient's desire to remain helpless and dependent outweighs the reality of his physical and mental limitations, or, conversely, when his desire to remain active and independent outweighs the reality of his physical and mental limitations.

Conflict

Conflict exists when the patient's conscious or unconscious thoughts, wishes, or feelings must be repressed because their expression would be unacceptable. It follows then that every "normal" medically ill patient is vulnerable to conflict between his psychosocially dictated need to adopt age- and phase-appropriate behavior and his physiologically dictated need to regress to an earlier mode of behavior, temporarily or permanently, in the service of maintaining physiological homeostasis.

Every individual, regardless of age, sex, or health status, unconsciously yearns at times to return to the passive, helpless, dependent state of childhood, when he was loved and cared for by mother. With maturity, this yearning conflicts with his fear of passivity; he equates this stance with helplessness, dependency, vulnerability, all of which may signify for him the loss of his vital self, that is, his intellectual, physical, and, in particular, his sexual capacities. Consequently, under "normal" circumstances, the individual strives—and is able—to keep his desire to be passive and cared for in check. However, with the onset of illness, there is a resurgence of this desire, which is reinforced by physical realities. The conflict between the desire to remain passive, on the one hand, and the self-condemnation evoked by overt manifestations of passivity, on the other, is then reactivated.

Many patients will be able to keep this conflict in abeyance. For some, however, the demand that they adopt a passive stance, to varying degrees and at intermittent stages of their illness, will have pernicious effects. In these individuals, this conflict may find expression in psychological symptoms—e.g., anxiety or depression—or in behavior that is deleterious to the patient's physiological status.

Object Relationships

The individual's capacity to relate to others, and, concomitantly, his ability to differentiate himself from others, will depend primarily on his constitutional endowment and his earliest experiences, which form the "bedrock of mental life."[16] His attitude and behavior toward others (and self) will be shaped by his early life experiences on two levels: His ongoing day-to-day experience with significant people in his environment, and the specific traumatic experiences to which he is exposed—e.g., the chronically rejecting attitude of a parent, the death of a parent or sibling, personal illness, injury, or hospitalization. And, inevitably, the individual's capacity to relate to others—and the quality of his relationships—will be further influenced by subsequent events, and, in particular, the onset of chronic illness. In that event, the most critical ingredient of his behavior may well become his relationship with his medical caretaker(s).

VEHICLES OF TRANSMISSION

If these basic psychological data are to be disseminated among the caretakers of the renal dialysis patient, it is essential to develop effective vehicles of transmission. We have discussed a medical–nursing–social service–teaching rounds format (ombudsman rounds) for the expansion of inservice curriculum training.[17]

The Ombudsman Rounds

It was decided that the key staff members of the renal dialysis team should meet weekly under the supervision of the assistant medical director of the unit and the liaison psychiatrist, to explore the psychosocial problems of individual patients, as well as medical issues and staff interactions. Patient interviews and staff interchange fostered a dynamic understanding of the mechanisms underlying the fears, anxieties, and hostility expressed by the patient to the staff, and, unintentionally, by the staff to the patient. These rounds were also designed to enable the staff participants to go beyond the routine aspects of patient care, and to deal with their feelings regarding their patients.

In accordance with the basic thrust of the ombudsman program, the participants select for presentation a series of dialysis patients who highlight psychosocial–medical issues and/or currently present urgent management problems, such as noncompliance, character trait disturbance (excessive passivity or activity), organic mental syndromes, depression, hypochondriasis, family reactions to medical illness, and the appropriate use of psychotropic medication. An informed consent is then obtained from the patient selected to join the staff at ombudsman rounds to discuss his reaction to his illness.

The staff meet weekly in the ombudsman's office.

Preinterview Discussion

Once the group has assembled, the ombudsman and/or liaison psychiatrist announces the name of the patient (who is not yet present), states the focus of the presentation, and invites comments from the staff regarding their perception of the patient, difficulties his care presents, and their impression of his reaction to his illness and the dialysis treatments. The group makes suggestions to the interviewer with regard to areas they would like explored.

The Interview

The patient is brought in, introduced to the group, and seated next to the interviewer. A typical greeting might be: "Good morning, Mr. M. How are you today? You remember we spoke to you about coming to this meeting and the staff is very grateful to you for coming. We would like to ask you a few questions." At the end of the interview, the patient is asked if he would mind if other staff members asked him some questions, or if he has questions of his own for the staff. The ombudsman and the liaison psychiatrist attempt to correct the patient's misconceptions as well as answer his questions, if they can. When the interview is concluded, the patient is thanked and told that the doctor will speak to him later.

Postinterview Discussion

The ombudsman or psychiatrist begins the discussion by asking the group what their responses were to the patient. Once these have been elicited, they attempt to formulate a psychosocial–medical understanding of the patient's behavior and to synthesize a treatment plan that encompasses all aspects of his care—psychological, social, and medical. Through such understanding, they hope to help the patient adapt to his illness and, at the same time, help the staff to adapt to the patient.

We try to have one of the members of the group study the patient, noting his reactions and learning how to deal with any problems or questions that may have emerged. At the postmeeting follow-up, the staff member attempts to assess ongoing patient behavior, further correct misconceptions, and provide psychosocial support in areas where the need for such support has become obvious from the rounds or follow-up. The accumulation of psychosocial data through later patient contacts permits confirmation of the accuracy of the original psychosocial–medical formulations, and, when indicated, further refinement of the therapeutic intervention.

It is our feeling that ombudsman rounds serve their function even if they only heighten the staff's awareness of the psychosocial reactions that are typically evoked by chronic illness. As a general rule, the staff's interaction during and after the patient interview creates a climate of interest in these factors. The liaison psychiatrist provides a synthesis of the psychosocial data that facilitates an interpretation of the patient's behavior.

The ombudsman rounds also provides a forum for discussion of the feelings that arise within the staff regarding such personal and professional issues as deciding whether a patient should be resuscitated in the event of a cardiac arrest, how the disoriented patient can best be cared for, and how to deal with the noncompliant patient. In short, ombudsman rounds create a setting in which anxieties, conflicts, and stresses in patients, as well as in the staff, can be examined—where the approach to medical care is enhanced by moving beyond physiological content to an awareness of the psychological needs of the patient and his caretakers.

Training and Funding

The effectiveness of the ombudsman conference hinges, in the final analysis, on the availability of a liaison psychiatrist who has been trained in the management of this patient population, and who has also been trained to disseminate his psycholo,gical knowledge and skills to the staff of the renal unit. The feasibility of assigning a liaison psychiatrist to such a unit is, unfortunately, economically determined.

In the renal dialysis satellite setting at Montefiore, we have overcome these impediments. We have established a liaison teaching unit described elsewhere[1] that incorporates measures which make it economically feasible to create a training position for a liaison psychiatric fellow (PGY-5 Trainee) who, as part of his training, provides psychological care on an ongoing basis for chronic renal patients. Specifically, under Public Law 92-603, Medicare payments of up to two hundred and fifty dollars ($250.00) per year are available for direct psychiatric consultation to all chronic renal dialysis and renal transplant patients who are eligible for Medicare for one year postsurgery, regardless of age (Table 1). In addition, Medicaid money may also be available for some patients. Under our program, in the past four years, we have been able to recruit liaison fellows* who have agreed that, in exchange for training in this subspecialty, they will provide direct services to a limited number of renal patients, the total fees generated by such services to be equivalent to the stipend customarily paid PGY-5 trainees (fellowship year), and to devote their remaining time to teaching psychological medicine to staff, e.g., ombudsman rounds, etc. (Table 2).

Essentially, we anticipated that in the course of the training year, intensive contact with this unique patient population (under supervision) would enable the liaison fellow to acquire the skills and knowledge necessary to provide these patients with adequate psychological care. We also anticipated that during this period, he would demonstrate these skills, to some extent, and disseminate this knowledge to the medical

*Drs. Samuel Langer, M.D., Daniel Blazer, M.D., J. Hampton Atkinson, M.D., Kathleen Degan, M.D., and Bodo Voldhardt, M.D.

TABLE 1

Funding Base

150 patients[a] × $250.00 =	$37,500/year
Liaison fellow's salary (for 20 h)	$12–14,000/year

[a]The number of patients treated in the satellite unit.

TABLE 2
Liaison Fellow's Teaching and Training Exercises

Exercise	Hours/week	
Patient contacts	10	
Ombudsman rounds	1	
Social worker conference	1	
Supervision with Director of		
Liaison Service	1	
Liaison Fellows' Workshop	1	
Medical psychology reading seminar	½	(18 sessions)
Psychobiology of human disease	½	(18 sessions)
Psychiatry grand rounds	1½	
Psychiatric research conference	1½	

caretakers with sufficient effectiveness, so that in time they would be able to function more autonomously in the psychological sector.

CONCLUSION

The end-stage renal patient exemplifies the plight of the chronically ill, machine-dependent ambulatory patient, who is inevitably faced with multiple psychosocial problems evoked by his illness and is currently deprived, by and large, of the services which would enable him to cope with these difficulties. If one concedes that the end-stage renal patient requires day-to-day emotional support of medical, nursing, and social work staff, one must also conclude that the standard psychiatric consultation method which provides psychiatric treatment on request, for those patients who present acute psychiatric disturbances, is grossly inadequate to this task.

In contrast, the liaison model attempts to ensure ongoing psychological care for these patients by enhancing the competence of the renal staff. The advantages of this model have not been sufficiently recognized primarily—but not solely—because of the erroneous notion that it is not financially feasible. In this chapter, I have outlined a plan for the financial implementation of this model under existing funding mechanisms. Once it had been established, the liaison teaching unit overcame impediments to the psychological care of the end-stage renal disease patient in the following way:

1. Patients were seen in the ambulatory medical setting, and even during renal dialysis procedures.
2. The nephrologist, the nurse, the social worker, and the technician formed a team that was taught the psychological reactions of the

medically ill, with the expectation that they themselves would, in time, deliver much of the mental health care required by this group.

3. The psychiatrist (liaison fellow) had "on the job training" under supervision, as well as ongoing didactic teaching, e.g., seminars, clinical presentations, etc. The bulk of the psychiatrist's salary was generated from fees for patient services, thus overcoming budgetary constraints that too often inhibited the provision of psychological support.

4. Psychological care was further enhanced by psychosocial–biological record-keeping which allowed for preliminary identification of those problems most commonly encountered in this group and concomitant emphasis on the management of such problems, e.g., suicide, noncompliance, sexual dysfunction, work inhibitions, reactions to stress, family response to illness, psychopharmacological complications, pain, organicity, etc.

Chronic renal patients are among those patients who are most in need of a supportive relationship with their medical caretakers, based on the caretakers' knowledge of the biological–psychological–social model of disease.[18] Given the availability of a teaching method which can ensure dissemination of the model—and thereby ensure adequate psychological care—for end-stage renal patients, and the means for the establishment of such a program, as outlined above, there can be no justification for depriving this patient group of the psychological services which are an essential part of their medical treatment.

REFERENCES

1. STRAIN, J. and LANGER, S. The liaison teaching unit: a funding mechanism for psychological care of the chronic renal patient (in preparation).
2. ABRAM, H. S. Psychiatric reflections on adaptation to repetitive dialysis. *Kidney International*, 1974, *6*, 67–72.
3. GLASSMAN, B. M. Personality correlates of survival in a long-term hemodialysis program. *Archives Gen Psychiatry*, 1970, *22*, 566–574.
4. DE-NOUR, A. K. and CZACZKES, J. W. Personality factors in chronic hemodialysis patients causing noncompliance with medical regimen. *Psychosomatic Medicine*, 1972, *34*, 333–334.
5. SAND, P., LIVINGSTON, G., and WRIGHT, R. G. Psychological assessment of candidates for a hemodialysis program. *Annals of Internal Medicine*, 1966, *64*, 602–610.
6. FOSTER, F. G., COHN, C. L., and MCKEGNEY, R. P. Psychobiologic factors and individual survival on chronic renal hemodialysis—a two year follow-up: Part I. *Psychosomatic Medicine*, 1973, *35*, 64–82.
7. VIEDERMAN, M. The search for meaning in renal transplantation. *Psychology*, 1974, *37*, 283–290.

8. VIEDERMAN, M. Adaptive and maladaptive regression in hemodialysis. *Psychology*, 1974, *37*, 68–77.

9. VIEDERMAN, M. Psychogenic factors in kidney transplant rejection: a case study. *American Journal Psychology*, 1972, *132*, 957.

10. ABRAM, H. S. The "uncooperative" hemodialysis patient: a psychiatrist's viewpoint and a patient's commentary. In N. B. Levy (Ed.), *Living or dying: adaptation to hemodialysis*. Springfield, Ill.: Charles C Thomas, 1974, pp. 50–61.

11. LEVY, N. B. Sexual adjustment to maintenance hemodialysis and renal transplantation: national survey by questionnaire: preliminary report. In N. B. Levy (Ed.), *Living or dying: adaptation to hemodialysis*. Springfield, Ill.: Charles C Thomas, 1974, pp. 127–140.

12. JACOBS, J., BERNHARD, M., DELGADO, A., and STRAIN, J. Screening for organic mental syndromes in the medically ill. *Annals of Internal Medicine*, 1977, *86*, 40–46.

13. GOTTLIEB, R., NAPPI, T., and STRAIN, J. The physician's knowledge of psychotropic drugs: preliminary results. *American Journal of Psychiatry*, 1978, *135*, 29–32.

14. CAPLAN, G. *Principles of preventive psychiatry*. New York: Basic Books, 1961.

15. STRAIN, J. J. and GROSSMAN, S. *Psychological care of the medically ill: a primer in liaison psychiatry*. New York: Appleton-Century-Crofts, 1975, pp. 1–10.

16. MAHLER, M. S., PINE, F., and BERGMAN, A. *The psychological birth of the human infant: symbiosis and individuation*. New York: Basic Books, 1975.

17. STRAIN, J., and HAMERMAN, D. Ombudsman–medical–psychiatric teaching rounds (ombudsman rounds). *Annals of Internal Medicine*, 1977, *80*, 550–555.

18. ENGEL, G. L. The need for a new medical model: a challenge for bio medicine. *Science*, 1977, *196*, 129.

4

Professional Stress and the Responses of Nurses Caring for Patients with Chronic Renal Failure

MARTHA O. LEONARD

INTRODUCTION

Nurses employed in nephrology units report that caring for patients with end-stage renal disease (ESRD) is an unusually stressful professional experience. Just how stressful this milieu is can be inferred from the apparent short tenure and high replacement rate among staff of dialysis and transplant units. Other observations reflecting this problem include the following:

- Some employers require a contractual commitment of at least two years employment in order to recover the high cost of training personnel for nephrology.
- Informal comments of peers indicate that nephrology is widely viewed as a depressing and unrewarding environment in which to work.
- There is reluctance to recruit and assign new or inexperienced nursing graduates to nephrology because of the acknowledged stressfulness of the area.
- Many dialysis and transplant services employ liaison psychiatrists whose primary responsibilities are the support and counselling of nursing and medical staffs who must interact with complex psychosocial needs of patients.

In each of these examples, the implication is that there are psychological stresses which are at least costly in terms of the delivery of effective

MARTHA O. LEONARD, M. N. • Clinical Nursing Specialist, Rogosin Kidney Center; and Department of Surgical Nursing, The New York Hospital, New York, New York.

nursing care, and worse, may be serious impediments to the utlization of nurses in therapeutic roles in nephrology services.

There appear to be two different derivations of this stress: (1) that which stems from particular characteristics of the ESRD patient population and (2) that which arises from conflicting role expectations of nurses and the other professionals who work with us in providing related services. A brief description of these different stressors may be useful in understanding the responses of nurses.

The major stresses experienced by nurses in ESRD care relate to the special needs of the patients and to particular characteristics of the ESRD population: (1) intensity of contact, (2) dependency, (3) chronicity, (4) consumerism.

INTENSITY OF CONTACT

The requirement for dialysis therapy two or three times a week brings the nurse and patient into close contact with each other as much as 15–20 h/week, for months and often years. These hours of relentless "togetherness" promotes the development of unusually close nurse–patient relationships. Usually, first names are used between patient and staff. Informality becomes an accepted norm. Gifts are exchanged. Staff–patient parties are held.

It is perhaps "natural" that a quasi-family environment develops within the dialysis unit. But, it is thereby also "natural" that this family will engage in squabbles, displays of affection, bursts of annoyance, interpersonal rifts, and even unrealistic emotional demands of the sort "love me, take care of me."

In general, there is little in the education or experience of most nurses which prepares them for the emotional consequences of this kind of professional involvement. How should the nurse respond when:

- a young man on dialysis asks her for a date?
- a wealthy patient of whom she is very fond buys her an expensive sweater for Christmas?
- her "favorite" patient becomes angry and accuses her of not "caring" when she misses a venipuncture?
- her usual morning patient tells another staff member that he wants her to "take over," because she is better at dialysis?
- an elderly patient lashes out in criticism because the nurse took too long at lunch and the patient needed her?

DEPENDENCY

It is often the "take care of me" expectations, given the unusually close staff–patient relationships, which result in very difficult dependency needs. Some ESRD patients adopt a sick role which dominates their lives. They accept being sick as an authorized abrogation of their normal responsibilities as adults, members of society, or participants in a family.

The corollary, of course, is that these patients also do not accept their responsibilities in the dialysis "family." Many express a sense of entitlement to the nursing staff in terms of excessive demands. Again, the nurse is confronted with such stressful situations as:

- the erascible woman who asks the nurse to do personal errands "on her way home"
- the sick child whose mother demands that the nurse meet every plaintive cry of the child
- the elderly patient who obviously isn't eating properly and who asks the nurse for a "loan" to buy food
- the helpless patient who insists that the nurse attend his every need essentially immediately

Nurses who may be quite skilled in managing such dependency problems over a short interval often find their own emotional resources and psychological independence worn down over months of exposure. They may resent the excessive demands and then feel guilty because they are unable to meet the needs expressed.

CHRONICITY

A nephrology service provides a peculiar cross between intensive care and chronic care. Patients who are medically stable for months suddenly enter a crisis period with some life threatening complication. The nursing staff might have perceived the patient as nearly "well," equating dialysis stability with good health. Even a significant change of therapy, such as a new kidney transplant, represents a renewal of the threat to life.

Nurses in transplant units are often told how well the patient was doing on dialysis, and how tragic the unsuccessful transplant was in disrupting the patient's life.

Nurses in dialysis units are also in an awkward environment; the patients are "chronic," "maintenance dialysis," "ambulatory care," or "self care." The emphasis is on teaching and rehabilitation. Yet, just out of psychological "sight" is the nurses awareness of the fragility of the patient's life. The nurse knows the statistics of mortality and morbidity, but those statistics don't seem to apply to *her* patient. Perhaps the statistics are obscured by relatively dependable dialysis technology, or by the success of the long-term survivors.

Still, as a stress point, this juxtaposition of health and illness, life and death, creates an always present tension for the nurse. How should she respond to the patient who:

- asks her opinion about getting married, is it "fair" to the prospective spouse?
- plans to postpone college until after he gets a transplant?
- tells the nurse she is worried about dying before her small children are grown?
- complains that a transplant has set him back years of progress?

CONSUMERISM

Patients with ESRD have often lived with their disease and its treatment for years. They are knowledgeable, critical, and frequently angry. In this era of unrestrained criticism of the entire medical establishment, nurses in nephrology find themselves not only on the front line, but somewhat unprotected. They must interact three times weekly with the same patients who may be verbally and emotionally abusive.

In a less critical mode, but still stressful, is the situation of experienced patient vs. inexperienced nurse. The new dialysis nurse soon finds that the patient's expectations are clearly stated, and the newcomer often has to "prove" herself.

AN ETHICAL DILEMMA

A slight variant of the patient stressor is the unresolved ethical issue common to many patient situations in nephrology.

Dialysis has been made available to all who suffer from ESRD. In the absence of selection limitations, a consequence of this policy has been to place some persons on dialysis for whom even a moderate standard of rehabilitation cannot be achieved. Nurses find themselves in painful conflicts because of their beliefs:

- dialyzing a patient with advanced cancer
- dialyzing the very old, senile patient from a nursing home
- dialyzing the patient who is totally uncooperative with the medical

regimen and who is a regular client of the emergency room because of self abuse

Even when nurses recognize the inherent impossibility of selection criteria, they still feel the stress of this apparent conflict. Professional frustration is a real source of stress.

ROLE CONFLICTS

The second grouping of stressors in nephrology are more generic, and therefore more difficult to assess. These have to do with the oft remarked gap between what nurses are taught about their roles in patient care, what they expect for themselves, and what the medical bureaucracy is prepared to endorse and/or support.

The education of nurses *exactly* emphasizes the role of the nurse as a primary therapist. Nurses are taught to value comprehensive care, including assessment of patient needs, care plans, patient and family teaching, counseling, and continuity of care. Standards of nursing practice require individualized care with a strong component of psychosocial support.

Unfortunately, a hospital bureaucracy in general, and ESRD services in particular, place a high premium on contradictory values such as technical efficiency, reduced staff/patient ratios, limited professional and more technical staff, and cost-saving equipment which requires that one nurse the equipment instead of the patient. There is little or no *operational* value assigned to more time consuming and less economical activities such as teaching, counseling, or one-to-one psychological support. In fact, Federal regulations mandate that only one nurse need be present during dialysis, regardless of the numbers or type of patients. The implication is that all direct patient care can be accomplished by technicians. Again, given the currrent pressure for cost containment, it is apparent to nurses that the real crunch in ESRD care will be to reduce the professional (i.e., nurses) components of patient care.

It should be clear that this is not just a paper conflict of values and attitudes. Our system for providing regular maintenance dialysis and outpatient medical supervision is based upon clear technical and economic priorities. The problems of facilitating adaptation to chronic illness are systematic fragmentation of responsibility and inadequate professional support, both of which compromise, if not preclude, primary therapeutic roles for nurses. The nurse is forced to sacrifice her own role conception for a less gratifying technical assignment. The nurse in dialysis may find that:

1. she is expected to dialyze more patients than she is able to do except in a highly efficient, i.e., technical way
2. she is assigned responsibility for supervision of technicians doing dialysis, but no direct patient care herself
3. there are very few opportunities for a relaxed, planned engagement of patients in teaching and/or counsling

Nephrology nurses have become accustomed to an internal role identification which is often called "expanded practice," or "advanced nursing practice." Many have participated in specialty training programs. The expectations they hold for themselves embrace the concepts of professional practice esteemed by nurses, not simply the application of technical skills which have been delegated by physicians.

It would appear that this collision of professional goals and identity is at the heart of much dissatisfaction in ESRD care, particularly as the impact of regulations and cost containment is felt.

ADAPTIVE AND MALADAPTIVE RESPONSES

Given these multiple sources of stress, nurses respond in a variety of ways—some of which can be seen as helpful to the process of professional adaptation and growth, and others of which are singularly maladaptive. Recognition and understanding of these responses may facilitate planning to meet staff needs.

Maladaptive responses are characterized by avoidance of conflict, emotional disengagement, and task orientation. Avoidance of conflict has been described by Kramer as a kind of "lateral arabesque." Nurses leave nephrology to return to school, to seek administrative routes of advancement, or to leave nursing altogether for industrial positions.[1:19] Emotional disengagement represents a decision not to get involved with patients, an attitude which cultivates indifference and boredom; e.g., "I really don't care, this is only a job." Task orientation is the functional approach to getting the job done by the most efficient and least demanding route possible; e.g., "I'll set up the machines, or give the medications, or take the vital signs." Each of these responses results in chronic frustration and anger as well as basic job dissatisfaction. As nurses invest less of themselves, the opportunity for effective development of therapeutic relationships is equally diminshed. Kramer describes this syndrome as "reality shock," a situation in which the aspirant professional perceives that many professional ideals and values are not operational and go unrewarded in the work setting.[1:ix]

The end result of these responses is the loss of effective personnel to care for ESRD patients. Nurses speak to each other of being "burned out," indicating that they feel unable to bring about significant change and are unwilling to endure their chronic anger and frustration. Notwithstanding the personnel consequences of these problems, Foster and McKegney have attempted to demonstrate a significant correlation of staff attitudes toward patients on chronic dialysis and length of patient survival.[2] The suggestion is that nurses who elect to stay in the field, but who feel strong negative or hostile feelings about their patients, may interact with patients in such a way as to diminish the patients cooperation with therapy.

Fortunately, there are other, more productive responses to the stress of caring for patients with ESRD, responses which can be cultivated when the problems are recognized and given priority. Examples include reorganization of the patterns of nursing practice to support primary nursing, the utilization of liaison psychiatric services, the development of patient/staff groups, and the establishment of meaningful (as opposed to *pro forma*) team conferences.

Primary nursing is a form of organization for the delivery of nursing care which emphasizes a responsible, accountable relationship of one patient to one specific nurse. This form of organization is especially useful in affording the nurse a sense of personal accomplishment of patient care objectives.[3]

The use of liaison psychiatric services has been particularly beneficial in this author's experience. The liaison psychiatrist must be accessible and must be involved in staff conferences to a degree sufficient to integrate his presence and his work with the nursing staff's.

Patient–staff group meetings have been successful in some settings, particularly outpatient hemodialysis units. Care must be taken that these group meetings do not disintegrate into social gatherings as opposed to opportunities for productive communication.

Meaningful team conferences are those which are characterized by mutual respect for the expertise of *all* members of the health team. A regular time must be set aside and given priority among the multiple demands for staff time. Physicians must be willing to hear about nursing objectives and conditions necessary to support those objectives. Nurses must be prepared to accept responsibility, accountability, and flexibility to carry out the medical plan of care as well as their nursing objectives. My objective in this conference is to encourage all participants to recognize the training and expertise of each professional discipline involved in ESRD care and to facilitate an environment in which maximum utilization of these skills is possible.

Caring for people with *chronic* disease demands a fresh look at the definition of patients' needs—which go far beyond the diagnosis and therapy of medical crises. Strauss, in his helpful book, *Chronic Illness and Quality of Life*, emphasizes that these needs include the following:

1. Prevention of medical crises
2. Control of symptoms
3. Management of problems related to therapy
4. Prevention of social isolation
5. Adjustment to changes in course of disease
6. Attempts to normalize lifestyle[4]

Clearly, there is a serious discrepancy between the organization of services provided the chronically ill (i.e., dialysis, transplantation) and the services our patients actually need to live successfully. Strauss states that this problem is traceable to the fact that these aspects of care are regarded as peripheral responsibilities of health personnel. He says,

> it is probable that until health personnel are genuinely responsible for the social and psychological aspects of giving care (as they are for the more purely medical and procedural aspects) there will be limited improvement in those aspects of care, except that which is effected fortuitously or temporarily because of an unusually skilled or compassionate or sensitive staff member.[4:137]

I would add to Strauss' conclusion that neither the responsibility assigned nor the compassion desired will be mobilized consistently over time by a staff which must focus so much of its energy in coping with professional stress.

These are problems of health care delivery, and these are real needs of patients with ESRD which can and should be addressed by the skills and interests of nurses. However, these needs are assigned low priority in our system of illness-related service. This gap in perceived needs and the consequent differences in role expectations among nurses, their employers, and other professionals generates considerable stress for nurses. The additional stresses attendant to the particular problems of the patient population further complicate and reduce the effective utilization of nurses in therapeutic roles. A strong commitment to improved communication and mutual respect between the health team members, and a realistic approach to dealing with these professional stresses will address these problems in a constructive way.

REFERENCES

1. KRAMER, MARLENE, and SCHMALENBERG, CLAUDIA. *Path to biculturalism.* Wakefield, Mass.: Contemporary Publishing, Inc., 1977.
2. FOSTER, F. GORDON, and MCKEGNEY, PATRICK F. Small group dynamics and survival on chronic hemodialysis, 1977–8, *International Journal of Psychiatry in Medicine, 8,* 105.
3. LEONARD, MARTHA. Health issues and primary nursing in nephrology care. *Nursing Clinics of North America,* 1975, *10,* 413–420.
4. STRAUSS, ANSELM. *Chronic illness and the quality of life.* St. Louis: The C.V. Mosby, 1975.

5

What's New on Cause and Treatment of Sexual Dysfunctions in End-Stage Renal Disease

NORMAN B. LEVY

There was relatively little systematic study of the sexual dysfunctions of patients with end-stage renal disease (ESRD) until 1972. Before then there was only speculation about the sexual functions of these patients, such as De-Nour who wrote in her 1969 paper on the psychological significance of urination.[1] There, the subject of phantom urination was discussed and the observation was made that men seemed to have more sexual difficulties after being on hemodialysis than before. In 1972, at a panel devoted to the psychological adaptation of patients on hemodialysis, Scribner concluded that concerning impotence, "No data on this are good, but about one-third report that they are quite normal, about one-third say they have decreased potency but have some sexual activity and about one-third report that they're completely impotent."[2]

In 1972 two studies were undertaken to investigate the prevalence of sexual dysfunctions in ESRD. Abram and his co-workers interviewed 32 male patients on hemodialysis, some of whom has received renal transplants[3] and I undertook a study of male and female hemodialysis and transplant patients by a nationwide questionnaire.[4] The results of both these studies pointed to marked deterioration in the sexual functions of patients undergoing hemodialysis, especially males. Decreased ability in the sexual functioning of patients who have received renal transplants was also shown, but much less so than experienced by those maintained on hemodialysis.

There has been a fair amount of discussion as to the cause of these

NORMAN B. LEVY, M.D. • Director, Liaison Psychiatry Division, and Professor of Psychiatry, Medicine, and Surgery, New York Medical College, Valhalla, New York. The answer to the question asked by the title of this chapter "What's New on Cause and Treatments of Sexual Dysfunctions in End-Stage Renal Disease?" is the subject of the September, 1978 edition of *Dialysis and Transplantation*.

sexual dysfunctions. Organic factors must play a role in a group of patients with impaired kidney functions, manifested by marked anemia and many complications of illness and its treatment. Psychological factors were incriminated on the basis of the finding of worsening in sexual functions as patients went from untreated uremia to treatment of hemodialysis. Depression, called the most common psychological complication of hemodialysis,[5] has been incriminated as a participating cause of some of the sexual dysfunctions.[6] Reversal in family role and the psychological significance of cessation of urination are factors primarily affecting men by its impairment of their sense of masculinity.

Recently there has been renewed interest in learning about the causes of the sexual dysfunctions of these patients. As to physical factors, in the male undergoing hemodialysis and to a lesser extent of those who are recipients of renal transplants, there is poor spermatogenesis with sperm counts markedly reduced and greatly diminished motility of sperm cells. There is also impaired testosterone secretion in most but not all of these patients. FSH levels are generally increased but not in all patients. LH levels are generally higher, with the usual formula that the higher the LH the better the testosterone secretion and the lower the LH the lower the amount of circulating testosterone.[7] The effect of hemodialysis on testicular function is one of diminishing sperm production and diminishing testosterone levels. However, hemodialysis seems to have no effect on either FSH or LH. In patients who are transplanted there is improvement in all these measures. In women, the progesterone levels are uniformly low. Women on hemodialysis are generally anovulatory and do not have periods. In general, hemodialysis does not improve either testicular or ovarian functioning. In summary, concerning endocrinological functioning in ESRD, the picture is a rather confused one. Worst of all there is great difficulty in correlating hormonal changes with sexual dysfunctions, especially in women.

However, there has been some recent work clarifying a bit or at least pointing in some directions as to physical reasons for the problems of sexual functioning in these patients. A group at the Veterans Administration Hospital in Washington under Antoniou in a pilot study of four male patients and four controls determined that zinc affects both the production of testosterone in males which was correlated in these patients with impotence.[8] Replacement therapy of zinc improved both testosterone levels and sexual functioning. However, this is a relatively small study, and only in males. It is important that there be further study of the effects of zinc on androgenic stimulation of prostatic tissue possibly resulting in prostatic hyperplasia or prostatic neoplasia.

The parathyroid seems to have a role in sexual functioning. Loew and his group studied sexual functioning in 33 dialysis patients and found

that 24 of them had varying degrees of impotence.[9] They found a significant correlation between the degree of impotence and the magnitude of
secondary hyperparathyroidism. Massry and his associates at USC discovered that the lowering of parathyroid levels was connected with both
improvement in testosterone levels and improved sexual functioning.[10]
Their work on only seven patients indicate that the parathyroid glands
may have an important role in sexual dysfunctions. Please note that these
studies only involve the male. Physical factors in the female, other than
the general effects of anemia and chronic illness, remain largely unknown.

As the differentiation between psychological and organic factors in
sexual dysfunctions of these patients, the work of Fisher and Karacan are
of help.[11,12] They discovered that in 80% of male patients, REM sleep is
associated with nocturnal penile tumescence. Therefore, by placing a
gauge around the base of the penis one can test the physical ability of the
penis to function properly by simultaneously placing electrodes indicating the presence of REM sleep. This study has been used by the
Karacan group on patients with ESRD. They discovered that there is a
reasonable decrease in the total amount of tumescence during sleep in
patients undergoing hemodialysis as opposed to age-matched controls.
Patients with transplantations have less of a dimunition.[13] These findings
favor the conclusion that organic factors play an important role in the
sexual dysfunctions of these male patients.

A number of other authors have worked on refined studies of the
epidemiology of sexual dysfunctions of patients with ESRD. Golden and
Milne studied 47 patients and reported significant decrease in the frequency of sexual interest and functioning in both males and females on
hemodialysis. With transplantation they found that there was no difference in the females. However, there was marked increase in interest in
sexual functioning of the males.

Finkelstein and Steele have attempted to correlate sexual functions
with affective states and psychological syndromes, especially that of
depression, using the KDS Scale.[14] They showed that there is a correlation between sexual problems and those patients on hemodialysis who
were most depressed.

As to the treatment of these sexual dysfunctions, the physical studies
point in a therapeutic direction. As mentioned, the use of zinc in those
males who have depletion in this element as well as the dimunition in
parathormone among those suffering from an excess of it, holds great
promise. However, the endocrinology of sexual dysfunctions in ESRD
required that much more work needs to be done to correlate hormonal
changes with actual sexual dysfunction.

With the aid of techniques of measuring nocturnal penile tumescence, there is a tool for the differentiation of psychological from organic in those patients in which such a distinction has importance.

As to the treatment of the psychological factors causing sexual dysfunction in these patients, depression seems to be well correlated with sexual dysfunction and its treatment with psychotherapeutic techniques including the use of antidepressants is warranted in many patients. Perhaps most promising and still quite under utilized are the application of modifications of Masters' and Johnson's techniques with patients with ESRD. There is a paucity of literature on this subject, with McKevitt[15] and Berkman[16] perhaps pointing the way. Their writings concerning their own limited experience seems to show that the use of behavioral techniques has an important role among selected patients.

There is no question that there is a dearth of information in this area altogether. However, with increased interest in both the clarification of the causes of sexual dysfunctions and the application of techniques addressed to their alleviation, there is great promise for progress in the near future.

References

1. De-Nour, A. K. Some notes on the psychological significance of urination. *Journal of Nervous and Mental Disorders*, 1969, *148*, 615–623.
2. Scribner, B. H. Panel: living or dying adaptation to hemodialysis. In N. B. Levy (Ed.), *Living or dying: adaptation to hemodialysis*. Springfield, Ill.: Charles C Thomas, 1974.
3. Abram, H. S., Hester, L. R., Epstein, G. M., and Sheridan, W. F. Sexual functioning in patients with chronic renal failure. *Journal of Nervous and Mental Disorders*, 1975, *160*, 220–226.
4. Levy, N. B. Sexual adjustment to maintenance hemodialysis and renal transplantation: nationwide study by questionnaire. *Transactions of the American Society of Artificial Int. Organs*, 1973, *19*, 138–143.
5. Lefebre, P., Nobert, A., and Crombez, J. C. Psychological and psychopathological reactions in relation to chronic hemodialysis. *Canadian Psychiatric Association's Journal* 1972, *17*, 9–11.
6. Levy, N. B. Psychological studies at the Downstate Medical Center of patients on hemodialysis. *Medical Clinics of North America*, 1977, *61*, 759–769.
7. Lim, V. S., Audetta, F., and Kathpalia, S. Gonadal dysfunction in chronic renal failure: an endocrinological review. *Dialysis and Transplantation*, 1978, *7*, 896–907.
8. Antoniou, L. D., Shalhoub, R. J., Sudhakar, T., and Smith, J. C., Jr. Reversal of uraemic impotence by zinc. *Lancet* 1977, *2*, 895–897.
9. Loew, H., Schultz, H., Busch, G. Klinische aspekte der impotenz mannlicher dauerdialyse-patienten. Med. Welt, 1975, *26*, 1651–1652.
10. Massry, S. G., Procci, W. R., and Kletzky, O. A. Impotence in patients with uremia: A possible role for parathyroid hormone. *Nephrology*, 1977, *19*, 305–310.
11. Fisher, C. O., Gross, J., and Zuch, J. Cycle of penile erection synchronous with dreaming (REM) sleep. *Archives of General Psychiatry*, 1965, *12*, 29–45.
12. Karacan, I., The effect of exciting pre-sleep events on dream reporting and penile erections during sleep. New York: Downstate Medical Center, Department of Psychiatry, 1965 (doctoral dissertation).

13. Karacan, L., Dervent, A., Cunningham, G., Moore, C. A., Weinman, E. J., Cleveland, S. E., Salis, P. A., Williams, R. L., and Kopel, K. Assessment of NPT as an objective method of evaluating sexual functioning in ESRD patients. *Dialysis and Transplantation*, 1978, 7, 872–877.

14. Finkelstein, F. O., and Steele, T. E. Sexual dysfunction and chronic renal failure: a psychosocial study of 77 patients. *Dialysis and Transplantation*, 1978, 7, 877–878.

15. McKevitt, P. Treating sexual dysfunction in dialysis and transplant patients. *Health and Social Work*, 1976, 1, 133–157.

16. Berkman, A. H. Sex counseling with hemodialysis patients. *Dialysis and Transplantation*, 1978, 7, 924–927.

6

Severe Psychiatric Disorder in Dialysis–Transplant Patients
The Low Incidence of Psychiatric Hospitalization

F. PATRICK MCKEGNEY, CARL RUNGE,
RICHARD BERNSTEIN, AND RAGON WILLMUTH

INTRODUCTION

Chronic hemodialysis and renal transplantation have become increasingly common modes of treatment for end-stage renal disease (ESRD). This increase has led to many reports about the psychological impact of these highly stressful treatment modalities. Abram and Buchanan[1] reviewed seven studies of transplantation patients, and found a wide range and a varying incidence of psychiatric syndromes. Penn and co-workers[2] reported that 32% of their 292 renal transplant patients had "significant psychopathology." Anxiety, depression, and delirium were the more common diagnoses in their population, of whom seven attempted suicide (2.3%). In a more recent study, Blazer et al.[3] found a 4.2% incidence of affective psychoses in 215 transplant patients, but did not report on any other psychiatric syndromes.

Suicide in dialysis patients was surveyed by Abram et al. in a 1971 mail questionnaire.[4] They reported 20 successful and 17 unsuccessful suicide attempts in a sample of 3478 patients (1.06%), which they interpreted as being a "significantly high incidence of suicidal behavior compared to that of the general population."[4] Kaplan De-Nour and Czaczkes found a 20% incidence of "psychotic complications" and a 27% incidence

F. PATRICK MCKEGNEY, M.D., CARL RUNGE, M.D., RICHARD BERNSTEIN, M.D., AND RAGON WILLMUTH, M.D. • Departments of Psychiatry and Medicine, University of Vermont College of Medicine, Burlington, Vermont. This work was supported in part by NIMH Training Grant MH No. 08052. This paper was presented, in part, at the Annual Meeting of the American Psychosomatic Society, Washington, D.C., March 31, 1978.

of "suicide risk" in a population on maintenance hemodialysis for between 6 months and 4 years.[5] Most of these and other studies have had methodologic problems, such as restricted samples, varying diagnostic criteria, and different treatment modalities. Further, there have been no studies of psychiatric disorder in a comprehensive dialysis–transplant program for ESRD.

The present study examines the incidence of severe psychiatric disorders in all persons seeking and receiving treatment for end-stage renal disease at one regional ESRD center over 6½-year period. For the purposes of this report, "severe psychiatric disorders" have been strictly defined as behavioral disturbances requiring admission to a psychiatric in-patient service. These are to be distinguished from the common, often severe but nonpsychotic, usually time-limited, and situationally-related stress reactions of patients undergoing hemodialysis or renal transplantation. The latter are managed at our institution by multidisciplinary team which includes a consultation–liaison psychiatrist.

The study includes all patients referred to the dialysis–transplantation program at the University of Vermont College of Medicine and Medical Center Hospital of Vermont (MCHV) from October, 1971, through December, 1976. Its sample size of 118 consecutive patients, followed for an average of more than three years, is quantitatively sufficient to support conclusions. Further, continued intensive involvement with all patients has facilitated follow-up data gathered by care-givers outside of our center and included in this report. Finally, the treatment team has remained virtually intact during the years of this study, ensuring the stability of the medical, including psychiatric, diagnostic, and treatment criteria used.

Program Description and Methodology

The University of Vermont Kidney Disease Treatment Center began in October, 1971, and offers outpatient and inpatient center hemodialysis, home dialysis training, and cadaveric and living-related kidney transplantation. Patients referred for treatment are initially seen with their families by a patient selection committee, consisting of the nephrologist director of the dialysis program (C.R.), the surgeon director of the transplant program, the psychiatrist consultant (F.P.McK.), the medical social worker assigned full-time to the program, and the head nurse of the dialysis nursing staff. The evaluation–selection process, which has been described more fully elsewhere,[6] does not use the presence or history of a psychiatric disorder to exclude a patient from treatment, because of our clinical experience, similar to that recently described by Streltzer et al.[7] Related factors, such as poor patient coping abilities and the absence of psychosocial supports, do influence the decisions about patient acceptance or rejection, or, more often, the choice of active treatment modality. It should be emphasized that the most significant factor determining treatment decisions is the biological status of the patient. Almost as important are the attitudes and feelings of the patient and family about dialysis and/or transplant. "Rejection" by the evaluation–selection process has been based almost as much upon major hesitation on the part of the patient and/or family as upon the patient's severely compromised physical condition.[6]

At initial evaluation, all patients are asked to complete several research instruments, data from which are not considered in the evaluation or treatment decision making process. One of these instruments is the Rotter Locus of Control Index, which is a 29 item (6 nonscored) instrument which taps generalized expectations of the source of one's control on an internal (low score)–external (high score) dimension.[8] The patients also complete the M–R sections of the Cornell Medical Index, containing 51 psychological symptom items with yes–no forced choice answers. A "cutting score" of four yes responses has been suggested, above which there is a strong probability of emotional disturbance.[9]

The treatment program is carried out by a team of approximately 25 persons, which includes all members of the selection committee. Much emphasis is placed on continuity of care and maximal staff communication about patients and their families. Two to three staff meetings are held per week in which patients are discussed, particularly those with acute problems. All efforts are made to follow patients closely over time and to continue contact with families even after patients' deaths.

The selection committee psychiatrist sees all patients and families in the initial evaluation and may see them later on informal rounds. He has little direct contact with patients in any ongoing care-giving role, but rather maintains close contact with the other staff, who have developed a basic competence is dealing with the wide range of major adjustment problems, organic brain syndromes, family crises, and other psychosocial difficulties. When dialysis–transplant patients need psychiatric hospitalization, they are usually admitted to the psychiatric unit at the Medical Center Hospital of Vermont. Good communication is possible with the two other general hospital psychiatric units in the region, with the result that the UVM dialysis–transplant program would be contacted if any of its patients were hospitalized. Records on all living patients are updated periodically, on the basis of either their frequent visits to the MCHV or contacts with their local medical care-givers.

Results

One hundred and twenty-one patients were evaluated for treatment of ESRD through December, 1976. Three patients were lost to follow-up, all having moved to other parts of the country. The remaining 118 patients are included in the present report. Characteristics of the 118 patients at the time of evaluation are shown in Table 1. The Rotter score is slightly skewed toward the external locus of control, consistent with the findings of others in ESRD populations.[10] The mean CMI score is well above the "cutting score" of 4, indicating a significant degree of emotional disturbance in this population of severely biologically ill persons. This is consistent with the findings of the independent initial psychiatric assessment, which diagnosed a characterologic or neurotic disorder in approximately 20% of the patients. Twenty percent of the patients were delirious at evaluation, usually related to their uremic state. In summary, these patients as a group were acutely and chronically quite ill biologically, were significantly emotionally disturbed, and were relatively financially impoverished, usually due to unemployment resulting from illness.

The survival status of these 118 patients according to their major treatment modality as of January, 1978, is shown in Table 2. The "conservative" treatment category includes patients who had not yet needed

Table 1
Patient Characteristics at Evaluation

Sex		
Male	65	
Female	53	
Mean age	43.4 years	SD = 16.9 (range 7–81)
Mean years, education	10.7 years	SD = 3.0
Mean income	$6,000/year	
Mean Rotter score	8.3	SD = 3.7
Mean CMI	7.4	SD = 6.9
Mean duration of renal disease	65 months	SD = 91.6 (range 1–588)
Diagnosis of renal disease		
Rapidly prog. glomerulonephritis	9	(8%)
Chronic glomerulonephritis	27	(23%)
Diabetes mellitus	12	(10%)
Polyarteritis-lupus erythematosus	8	(7%)
Polycystic kidney disease	11	(9%)
Congenital kidney disease	8	(7%)
Chronic pyelonephritis	9	(7%)
Other	13	(11%)
Unknown etiology	21	(18%)

active treatment of ESRD. The 16 dead patients include 3 who declined dialysis and transplant, 10 who were "rejected" by the selection committee, and 3 who died of other causes before treatment for renal failure was necessary. The high death rate among this group of patients attests to the highly stressful nature of this disease–treatment situation.

The mean length of psychiatric follow-up of patients from time of evaluation to death or January, 1978, was 36 months. During this time, ranging from 13 to 78 months, 6 of the 118 patients required psychiatric hospitalization. Given the 40% incidence of psychiatric diagnoses made at initial evaluation, the highly stressful nature of the illness–treatment course, and findings in other studies,[2,3,5] this frequency of psychiatric hospitalization is considered to be surprisingly low. Brief case reports of these 6 patients, summarized in Table 3, will be followed by a discussion of the implications of these findings.

Case Histories

Depression Associated with Physical Illness

A.B. was a 36-year-old male who died following a long and complicated medical course. Diagnosed as having a cerebral hemangioblastoma at age 25, he later developed glomerulonephritis from an infected ventriculoatrial shunt which had been placed to treat the hydrocephalus caused by the tumor. Renal failure began four years after the initial craniotomy. After two years of center and home dialysis, A.B. had a cadaveric kidney transplant, by which time he was legally blind from optic atrophy. Two years after transplantation severe peripheral vascular disease necessitated amputation of his left leg. Death was caused by septicemia from a stump infection.

Psychiatric hospitalization occurred approximately one year after the start of dialysis and was precipitated by A.B.'s cutting his shunt in a suicide attempt. His situational depression was caused by A.B.'s multiple disabilities compounded by a character structure marked by poor impulse control and chronic low self-esteem. Intensive therapy in the hospital emphasized limit setting, his worth to others, and others' concern for him. Antidepressant and anxiolytic agents were also used. This treatment approach was continued by the dialysis team for the duration of the patient's life.

Dialysis Dementia

C.D. was diagnosed as having rapidly progressive glomerulonephritis at the age of 52, prior to which she had been in good health. Soon thereafter, she began dialysis first at hosptial and then at home, which continued for the next three years. Her course was complicated by hypertension, anemia, secondary hyperparathyroidism with severe osteodystrophy, and progressive en-

TABLE 2
Patient Survival Status as of January 1, 1978[a]

Treatment modality	Alive	Dead
Conservative	3	16
Home or center dialysis alone	23	28
Dialysis p̄ transplant failure	10	8
Functioning transplant	22	8
Total	58	60

[a]Mean follow-up 36 months (range 13–78 months).

TABLE 3
Psychiatric Admissions

Patient	Sex	Age	Rx[a]	Status (mos.)[b]	Major problems
A.B.	M	36	CD, HD, TX	dead (48)	1. blindness 2. asocial personality disorder 3. depression with suicide attempt 4. severe vascular disease
C.D.	F	55	HD, CD	dead (36)	1. dialysis dementia 2. hyperparathroid osteodystrophy 3. intractable pain 4. depression with self-exsanguination
E.F.	F	19	CD, TX	alive (33)	1. sudden psychosexual maturation 2. family disruption 3. steroid medication 4. paranoid psychotic reactions
G.H.	M	29	CD, TX, CD	dead (30)	1. diabetes mellitus (juv.) 2. neuropathy 3. blindness 4. poor impulse control 5. inadequate social support system 6. decision to no longer live
I.J.	F	48	HD, CD	alive (20)	1. poor impulse control 2. inadequate social support system 3. major marital disruption 4. suicidal ideation 5. conversion psychotic reaction
K.L.	M	37	CD, TX	alive (40)	1. mental retardation 2. dependent personality disorder 3. interference with treatment 4. refusal to leave hospital

[a]Rx, in temporal sequence; HD, home dialysis; CD, center dialysis; TX, renal transplantation.
[b]Status in months after evaluation until death or 12/77.

cephalopathy. She died by self-induced exsanguination through her shunt while in an extended care facility at the age of 55.

The onset of depression was noted approximately one year prior to the patient's death. Mild at first, with only a few neurovegetative signs, it progressed steadily despite antidepressant medication, and was complicated by the encephalopathy. When she was admitted to the psychiatric unit seven months prior to her death she was confused, wished to die, and had undergone a marked personality change. There was improvement in mental state with significant increase in function during hospitalization, but the patient remained discouraged and did not want to return home. One month before she died, again severely depressed, agitated, and confused, she was admitted to a nursing unit. At the time of the patient's death, her family and the dialysis team were reevaluating the desirability of continued treatment.

Posttransplant Psychosis

E.F. is a 20-year-old female whose renal failure first began when she was 11, which severely compromised her biological and psychosexual maturation. She received a kidney transplant from an older sibling when she 17, which has functioned quite well. There have been, however, four psychotic episodes since transplantation, two of them requiring hospitalization.

Her first psychotic episode occurred three weeks posttransplant when steroids were being manipulated, which six weeks later developed into a full-blown paranoid psychosis requiring psychiatric hospitalization. Both the steroids and significant intrapsychic conflicts, related to sudden pubescence, contributed to her decompensation. Phenothiazines and psychotherapy brought about a rapid improvement. One year later the patient was again hospitalized because of increased anxiety and paranoia, at a time when her steroid dosage was being increased and her parents' marriage was deteriorating. A fourth episode, not requiring hospitalization, occurred two years after transplantation. She is currently being maintained on imipramine and outpatient psychotherapy.

Diabetes and Decision to Die

G.H. was 29 years old at the time of his death. Forty-eight hours before his death he elected to discontinue insulin and hemodialysis and to die from the consequences of his diabetes and renal failure.

Diabetes mellitus was diagnosed at age 9. In addition to the diabetic nephropathy which led to renal failure and hospital hemodialysis at age 26, he had severe and progressive retinopathy and neuropathy with symptoms of impotence and chronic extremity pain. After bilateral nephrectomy, a cadaveric transplant at age 27 was immediately rejected. Home dialysis was not advisable because no family member was considered appropriate as a helper, and finances precluded hiring an aide. As his incapacity increased he became irascible and emotionally labile. His relationships with his wife and two children seriously deteriorated. He was forced to stop work because of his failing vision and could no longer drive himself the two hours to center dialysis.

Admission to the psychiatry service followed his threatening to shoot his wife and children during an episode of enraged frustration. He was depressed but not psychotic, and he articulated well the very difficult reality issues confronting him. In couples' therapy his wife expressed reluctance to have him come home immediately. The psychiatric staff strongly supported his making a decision to live or to die, an issue he had discussed extensively with the dialysis staff over many months. G.H. was assured that he would not be abandoned should he choose not to go on living. In the three weeks of his psychiatric hospitalization he vacillated about this decision but one morning decided he would not take insulin nor would he accept further dialysis. Several meetings with the psychiatric and medical staff and family conferences were held. The patient remained adamant in his decision to die, with the eventual concurrence of all persons involved. He requested transfer to the renal unit, where he received adequate pain medication. In the presence of his family and some of the dialysis staff, G.H. died 24 hours after transfer.

Chronic Psychosocial Turmoil

I.J. is a 48-year-old married woman with seven children. She developed renal failure due to chronic pyelonephritis, and at age 46 was begun on home hemodialysis, helped by her husband. Six months after beginning dialysis she required psychiatric hospitalization because of "paranoid" ideas about the husband's "infidelity," severe anxiety, and threats of suicide.

Psychiatric inpatient evaluation revealed longstanding marital discord but no severe psychiatric illness in the patient or her family. Four of her own seven children plus her son's fiancee and their infant child lived with the patient at the time of her psychiatric admission. The home atmosphere was described by everyone as noisy and chaotic. When the husband acknowledged his wish to separate from his wife and family, Mrs. J. was panicked by this threatened separation and talked of pulling out her A-V shunt. Within a few days, however, the husband reversed his position and proclaimed his intention of continuing to live with his wife and to perform her home dialysis. Six weeks after her discharge, the husband did leave the patient for another woman. Mrs. J. made a suicidal gesture, taking 400 mg of Mellaril, but was not readmitted to the psychiatry service. She continued to be seen as an outpatient by a psychiatric social worker and was placed on in-center hemodialysis. A year after hospitalization she had a psychotic episode.

Reluctance to be Well

K.L. is a 37-year-old mentally retarded, single man. In his late twenties he required multiple catheterizations for urinary retention of unknown, perhaps psychogenic, origin. At age 34 he began center hemodialysis for his chronic renal failure. After six months of dialysis he had a successful transplant of his brother's kidney. Five months following transplant he was admitted to the medical ward for evaluation of increasing renal failure, but no significant transplant rejection was found. The patient had taken his immuno-suppressant drugs unreliably, seemed to be voluntarily retaining large volumes of urine, and showed great reluctance to leave the hospital. Transfer to the psychiatric service was initiated in order to better assess and manage his lack of compliance with treatment and his increasing dependency on the hospital. His family had become angry and frustrated by what they believed to be the patient's deliberate efforts to gain continued attention by remaining ill.

On the psychiatry service he was placed on a behavior modification program. After a period of considerable resistance, K.L. began to increase his fluid intake and urinary output. His family was taught to use money to reinforce his taking immunosuppressant drugs and maintaining an adequate intake and output. Discharge home was accomplished only after several attempts by the patient to convince the staff that he was too "unreliable" to survive outside of a hospital. Continued outpatient psychiatric care has been provided in his local community.

Discussion

Three of the six patients requiring psychiatric hospitalization during this 6-year period presented with common psychiatric syndromes. C.D. had a psychotic reaction associated with a progressive organic brain syndrome. Her wish to die in the face of overwhelming physical and social disaster should, however, be distinguished from the suicidality of most psychiatric patients. Parenthetically, three other patients in our program with a clearly defined "dialysis dementia" syndrome[11] did not require psychiatric hospitalization. Their behavior was compatible with their being admitted to the renal unit for discontinuation of dialysis because of their progressively deteriorating physical condition. I.J. was admitted because of an inability to adapt successfully to psychosocial turmoil. The fact that she was on dialysis, assisted by her husband, only complicated the situation. A.B. had a depressive reaction in large part related to his physical illness, which interfered with his usual mode of coping with life stress.

Two other patients were rather different from the usual psychiatric admission, in that their psychological disturbance was in reaction to successful renal transplantation. E.F.'s transplant was followed by a rapid physical and psychosocial maturation compressed into three months, after a life of chronic illness and delayed psychosexual development. This stress, plus the biological effects of the steroid medication, led to her psychotic disruption. K.L. could not adapt to a "well role" after a life which had centered around hospitals, and this led him to seriously interfere with his medical regimen.

The sixth patient, G.H., was similar to the usual psychiatric admission in that he needed a separation from home and family, and close interaction with a "neutral" psychiatric staff. However, what made him so "nonpsychiatric" was the emotion-laden but rational decision he needed to make about continuing to live in the face of a deteriorating physical and psychosocial situation. While he had initially been given a diagnosis of a character disorder, he did not have a defined psychiatric illness warranting his psychiatric hospitalization. His threat to kill his family was not substantial, but rather a cry for decision making "time and space."

Our finding that only 5% of the patients followed for an average of more than three years required psychiatric hospitalization seems to be at variance with the incidence of psychotic reactions, suicide risks, and other psychiatric disorders reported in the literature.[2-5] In the opinion of the program staff, several factors seem to have contributed to this finding. First, a consultation–liaison psychiatrist has been an integral member of the dialysis–transplant staff from its inception, spending six to eight hours per week actually working in the program. This psychiatrist has not himself provided care to patients as an alternative to psychiatric hospitalization for psychological disturbances. Rather, he has worked with the staff in identifying and dealing with patients' coping problems at an early stage, actually beginning with the evaluation process. This process may have forestalled the development of behavior disruptions sufficient to warrant hospitalization. There have been a few occasions when patients were admitted to the renal inpatient unit for psychological problems, usually epxressed in somatic symptoms. However, few psychiatric units would have viewed these patients as appropriate admissions. Thus, the apparent incidence of severe psychiatric disorder in this patient population has not been artifically lowered by alternatives to psychiatric hospitalization.

Another major factor in the low incidence of psychiatric disorder seems to be that of staff competence and cohesion. The UVM dialysis–transplant program has expanded greatly over the years, as the patient population has increased. Despite the usual problems of size and the many stresses upon the staff associated with the nature of the patient problems,[12] there has been a generally high level of staff morale, as reflected by almost no staff turnover in six years. Strong physician involvement, frequent staff meetings, a policy of openly discussing staff feelings and problems, a considerable degree of socialization, and even a staff softball team, have contributed to this morale.

When these six patients were hospitalized on the psychiatric unit, the renal staff worked very closely with the inpatient psychiatry staff, helping them cope with the biological factors in the situation. The renal staff also worked with these patients and their families in the role of an extended family, clearly emphasizing that they were ready, after the patient's discharge, to resume their comprehensive care of the patient's and family's problems. Indeed, the renal staff's availability and holistic concern may be the most important factor in the paucity of severe psychiatric disturbances.

Our finding of a relatively low incidence of severe psychiatric problems in patients facing major biological illness and psychosocial disruption, many of whom with preexisting psychopathology, raises a significant question about the role of environmental stress in the development of the classical severe psychiatric syndromes. Two of the six patients (C.D., E.F.) had severe organic brain syndromes contributing to their psychiatric hospitalization. E.F. was the only patient in the group of six who manifested delusional thinking.

Our report is not a controlled study, and these conclusions have been drawn by the program's staff. However, we feel that these findings in a mean 3-year follow-up of 98% of a total population of 121 patients with end-stage renal disease warrants some conclusions: the need for psychiatric hospitalization in these patients is low; the reasons for these hospitalizations are quite varied; and the actual incidence of severe psychiatric disorders in this population is much lower than reported by others. The reasons for these findings seem to be: the development of a competent, cohesive, and dedicated dialysis–transplant treatment staff; the inclusion of a consultation–liaison psychiatrist with patient care, team development and group maintenance functions; and a treatment program philosophy which is continuous and comprehensive, for all problems and all family members, and not limited in time.

ACKNOWLEDGMENTS. The authors wish to express appreciation for the efforts of Roger Foster, M.D., Alice Wynne, R.N., Cathy Brown, M.S., and all of the other members of the UVM Dialysis–Transplant Program and especially to Ms. Donna Heuser.

REFERENCES

1. ABRAM, H. S., and BUCHANAN, D. C. The gift of life: a review of the psychological aspects of transplantation. *International Journal of Psychiatric Medicine,* 1976–1977, 7, 153–164.
2. PENN, I., BUNCH, D., OLENIK, D., and ABOUNA, G. Psychiatric experience with patients receiving renal and hepatic transplant. In P. Castelnuovo-Tedesco (Ed.), *Psychiatric aspects of organ transplantation.* New York: Grune and Stratton, 1971.
3. BLAZER, D. G., PETRIE, W. M., and WILSON, W. P. Affective psychoses following renal transplant. *Disorders of the Nervous System* 1976, 37, 663–667.
4. ABRAM, H. S., MOORE, G. L. and WESTERVELT, F. D. Suicidal behavior in chronic dialysis patients. *American Journal of Psychiatry* 1971, 127, 1199–1207.
5. KAPLAN DE-NOUR, A., and CZACZKES, J. W. The influence of patients' personality on adjustment to chronic dialysis. *Journal of Nervous and Mental Disorders,* 1976, 162, 323–333.
6. McKEGNEY, F. P. The patient's role in beginning and continuing maintenance hemodialysis. *Proceedings of the 5th International Congress on Nephrology* (Mexico, 1972), Vol. 3, Karger-Basel: 1974, 220–225.

7. Streltzer, J., Markoff, R. A., and Yano, B. Maintenance hemodialysis in patients with severe pre-existing psychiatric disorders. *Journal of Nervous and Mental Disorders*, 1977, *164*, 414–418.
8. Rotter, J. B. Generalized expectancies for internal versus external control of reinforcement. *Psychology Monographs*, 1966, *80*, 1–28.
9. Brodman, K., Erdman, S. J., and Wolff, H. G. The cornell medical index health questionnaire, Manual. New York: Cornell University Medical College, 1956.
10. Milatt, S. R., and Allain, A. Personal correlates of renal dialysis patients and their spouses. *Southern Medical Journal* 1974, *67*, 941–944.
11. Editorial: dialysis dementia. *British Medical Journal, 6046*, 1976, 1213–1214.
12. Kaplan De-Nour, A., and Czaczkes, J. W. Emotional problems and reactions of the medical team in a chronic hemodialysis unit. *Lancet*, 1968, *2*, 987–991.

7

The Role of the Chaplain as a Member of the Renal Dialysis Kidney Transplant Team

RAYMOND B. ANDERSON

The purpose of this chapter is to discuss the role of the hospital chaplain in the care of the renal dialysis and kidney transplant patient. The material for this paper is primarily drawn from my experience as a member of the renal dialysis team of the New England Deaconess Hospital. The discussion of the chaplain's role will be illustrated by a case study involving three patients, their families, and the hospital staff.

Initially, I feel it is important to provide some underlying assumptions about ministry in the hospital and the meaning of pastoral care.

> Pastoral Care may be defined as a religious ministry to individual persons in dynamic relationships arising from insight into essential needs and mutual discovery of potentialities for spiritual growth. A pastor is essentially one who cares for persons. First in a sense of affectionate concern and second in the active service of spiritual needs . . . The pastor personalizes his attention to the needs of individuals seeking to understand what life means to each one. . . .[1]

The tools of pastoral care are drawn from the disciplines of theology, psychology, and sociology.

The role of the hospital chaplain is to apply, develop, and integrate these basic assumptions into his ministry within the institutional setting. In the past decade the institutional chaplaincy has developed into an exacting and demanding discipline which requires posttheological training, and in a growing number of institutions certification by agencies such as the College of Chaplains of the American Protestant Hospital Association, and the Catholic Hospital Association.

As a hospital chaplain, I bring to my work and this paper a number of

---

RAYMOND B. ANDERSON, M. DIV. • Fellow, College of Chaplains, A.P.H.A.; Staff Chaplain, Department of Pastoral Care, New England Deaconess Hospital, Boston, Massachusetts.

underlying assumptions about what the chaplain does and who he/she represents. These assumptions will gain importance as I discuss my role as the "Renal Chaplain." My first assumption is that the hospital chaplain is the person, male or female, who is designated by the hospital to provide pastoral care to the patients and the staff within that community. The chaplain, if he is to be effective must understand his ministry in an ecumenical perspective. The chaplain is called to minister to the needs of the hospital community, the patient, the patient's family, and the staff irrespective of his religious affiliation. In ministering to people the chaplain respects their religious traditions (or lack of tradition) and thus is not out to convert or "give religion" to those with whom he is called to minister. As a chaplain I must recognize the fact that the majority of my ministry may occur with people of religious faiths different from my own. This fact is substantiated by Carey in a recent study entitled *Hospital Chaplains, Who Needs Them?* "Eighty-five percent of the patients report that having a chaplain *of some faith* available to them at all times is either of moderate or of great value."[2]

It has been my own experience that, except for the sacramental ministries, as the level of emotional stress increases, the importance of the denominational affiliation of the chaplain decreases. This fact has implications for the chaplain's role as a member of the renal team, in that the the chaplain or hospital staff need not be overly concerned or expect that ministry cannot occur unless patient and chaplain are of the same, or similar, faith traditions. Carey's study also showed that the medical staff are generally receptive to having chaplaincy available regardless of denomination.

> Eighty-seven percent of nurses and seventy-six percent of doctors placed *great* value on the services of the chaplaincy . . . only about one-third (of the staff) said that it was of great importance to have a chaplain of the same faith as the patient.[2]

Thus, it would seem that the quality of care provided is more important than the chaplain's religious denomination.

The second major assumption that I bring to this paper is that the chaplain represents not only religious faiths, or even a particular denomination, but in a very real sense the chaplain represents and incarnates God. This "incarnational" understanding is based on the transference, whether positive or negative, which occurs between the patient and the chaplain. Thus, the effectiveness of the chaplain in ministering to a patient may be determined by the content of such transference and the chaplain's understanding of, and ability to use, the transference. Through this transference a relationship may occur which is different from the relationship which occurs between patient and other members of the renal dialysis team. This relationship is different because of how the chaplain views his role and how the patient understands that role.

First let us look at the chaplain's self-perception. "The role of the chaplain in the care of the patient is one of 'being' with instead of advising, choosing, or doing."[3] The chaplain's stance with the patient is that of an active listener whose purpose is to address the needs of the patient on the patient's terms. Thus, the chaplain brings neither tools, such as medicine, nor task, such as treatment. Instead, the chaplain brings a blank prescription pad which in a sense is filled in by the patient rather than by the doctor. This understanding of his/her role places the chaplain in a unique position among hospital staff. The chaplain brings to the patient the task of "being" with the patient in his crisis. Listening and being present are his primary tasks. To be sure, at times there may be overlap in this role with other members of the team, especially the social worker and the psychiatrist. And yet our experience shows that there is room for us to work both together and separately with the patient in complimentary ways.

The patient may experience the chaplain as different from the other members of the hospital staff. The chaplain may be seen by the patient as being in, but not of, the hospital community by the patient and his or her family. Because the chaplain is placed in this position, the patient may risk the expression of certain feelings, hopes, and requests to the chaplain that he/she might not necessarily express to other members of a caring team. The patient often sees himself in the position of total dependency upon the doctor, surgeon, and nursing staff. This is perhaps acutely true for the dialysis and pretransplant patient. With such dependency it is easy to understand why the patient may fear being truly honest with the medical team, especially if such honesty is critical of the care being received. Since the patient experiences the staff chaplain as not being part of the medical team, there is less dependency and thus less risk involved in being honest. Thus, the patient experiences the chaplain as an advocate, as a person he can confide in about the frightening emotional and spiritual stresses experienced because of illness. If the chaplain is to remain effective and trusted by both the patient and the staff, it is important for him to retain autonomy within the hospital setting by not being the one who must defend either the hospital or the patient.

If the patient is struggling with such issues as hope, the meaning and purpose of life, anger, or fear of dying he/she will very likely choose to discuss these "religious" issues with the chaplain. Thus, although a patient may or may not consciously espouse belief in God, he may raise these issues to consciousness in the presence of the chaplain.

> As a minister of God, the chaplain will deal with dying, and death, living and life's meaning, and all this is within the context of the patient's own reaction and choices. Leading his theological and sacramental ministry into the concrete, personal life situations of the particular patient is a delicate process demanding creative effort in a spirit of service.[3]

At the New England Deaconess Hospital, the Dialysis Unit is a five-bed acute care unit located on one end of a medical/surgical floor. All five beds are in one room with no isolation provisions. Because of the smallness of the unit, there tends to be a lack of privacy. Thus, unless the person receiving dialysis is an outpatient, most pastoral visiting occurs with the patient back in his/her own room. The dialysis unit is operated on a two-shift basis, Monday through Friday, from 7:30 a.m. to 11:30 p.m. The unit operates on Saturday from 7:30 a.m. to 3:30 p.m. Time is made available between shifts for staff meetings and staff education. The normal patient census is between 16 and 20, of whom approximately 20% are outpatients. The dialysis unit is operated in such a way that once a patient is medically stable, he is referred to a chronic unit close to home. Yet, there is a continual number of chronic dialysis patients at the Deaconess Unit because of a backup at local chronic units, problems with transportation, or insufficient funding.

The other 80% of the patients are in the hospital for various medical/ surgical reasons, or for kidney transplantation. Approximately 50% of the patients being treated are transplant candidates. Of the total population of the dialysis patients at the Deaconess Hospital 80% are diabetics suffering from all of the related complex psychosocial and medical problems. The Deaconess Dialysis Unit provides acute care and hospitalization coverage for approximately seven chronic facilities in the Massachusetts and Rhode Island area. The unit is staffed by seven nurses, six full-time and one part-time, and a resident nephrologist. The nurses are responsible for patients and hospital staff education regarding dialysis and transplantations, as well as direct patient dialysis.

The treatment team (consisting of two separate nephrology teams and two separate surgical teams) which cares for the renal patient includes five nephrologists, four surgeons, our dialysis-unit head nurse, the dialysis-unit teaching nurse, a staff psychiatrist who works with the team on a part-time basis, the renal dietician, the renal social worker who is also responsible for one hospital floor involving approximately 28 patients plus previous clients, the physical therapist, and the chaplain, who is responsible for two other floors of approximately 70 patients plus returning patients with whom a pastoral relationship has been previously developed.

The Department of Pastoral Care's relationship with the renal team has evolved over a six-year period. The team functions in a number of ways. It meets approximately three Thursdays out of the month. The first hour of the meeting is used to discuss the psychosocial aspects of patient care. During this time, a patient's case is presented by one of the members of the team, usually the psychiatrist, social worker, or the chaplain. This meeting is often attended by other interested members of the hospital staff who have had contact with the patient and who feel they may have something important to offer, or who may be able to learn from the input of the other team members. During the second hour the nephrologist and surgeons present cases which they feel they need to discuss for medical and/or other reasons. It is also at this time that the names of prospective transplant patients are discussed.

Both of these meetings provide the chaplain the opportunity to initiate involvement through consult and informal referral with new or previously unfamiliar patients. The chaplain also attends a midweek teaching round for the dialysis unit nurses taught by the unit nephrologist. The teaching rounds, as well as the kidney rounds, will at times include medical information that may not be directly helpful nor necessary for the chaplain to know in order to provide good pastoral care. Yet, in a nonspecific way, these rounds provide the chaplain with a growing wealth of knowledge which adds to his understanding of the effects of kidney failure upon the patient and the patient's family from both a medical and emotional perspective. It is also this chaplain's assumption that contact with and interest in the work of the other members of the renal team who are attending these rounds is helpful in developing a trusting relationship. Because chaplains frequently are not part of the health care teams, they need to develop meaningful working relationships with the other members of the hospital team if they expect to be integrated into the patient's care plan.

Another essential role that the chaplain can perform in the setting of the dialysis and kidney transplant rounds in order to provide good patient care is to use the raw data which is presented and place over this material what might be called "a pastoral care grid." The chaplain can then examine this new material which has been filtered through the discipline of pastoral care and subconsciously ask such questions as: What does it do to a man's dignity and meaning of life when he is disabled at the age of 37 and has a wife and three children to support? What happens to a young diabetic's hope and belief in justice if he has followed his diet faithfully and taken insulin as directed and yet finds his health continues to disintegrate? Dr. Paul W. Pruyser, a Clinical Psychologist in the Menninger Foundation, in his book, *The Minister as Diagnostician,* presents the thesis that "Pastors, like all other professional workers, possess a body of theoretical and practical knowledge that is uniquely their own . . ."[4] He states that such understanding may be helpful because "A patient's religious views, belief system and value orientation are important for what it allows us to state about his felt personhood and conflict."[4] The chaplain on the renal team has the opportunity, then, to grow in his own knowledge of the patient and his problem, and at the same time provide insight and information to the other members of the team in order to enhance the understanding and care of the renal patient.

The following pages of this paper will focus on the chaplain's ministry to three patients, the patient's family, and the hospital staff who cared for the patient.

The first patient is a female in her mid-30s, married with three children, and with a history of juvenile onset diabetes mellitus. This woman, whom we shall call Nancy, was admitted to the hospital for the purpose of receiving a kidney from her father. My first contact with Nancy occurred during a presurgical call on the evening before her transplant surgery. Nancy had been on dialysis for a short period of time prior to her surgery. At the time of her surgery, Nancy was a patient on one of my assigned floors, and, thus, along with the renal social worker, I continued to visit her on a regular basis in order to provide her with emotional support. About three weeks after her transplant surgery, I was approached by the head nurse of the Dialysis Unit and the head nurse of Nancy's floor and asked if I would become primarily responsible for providing emotional support to Nancy, since the renal social worker was leaving the hospital. Although the new renal social worker could have followed through on this referral, the nursing staff felt that I had already established a trusting relationship with the patient. Nancy, as well as those responsible for her care, felt that it was important for her to have continuity in her relationship with someone from the hospital staff. Nancy was hospitalized for an extended period of time and since the Deaconess is a teaching hospital, Nancy soon began to experience a number of losses as the medical residents would move off of her floor during their rotation, plus the loss of her social worker whom she had grown to know and trust.

Although she continued to receive good medical care, Nancy began to experience a growing sense of emotional stress which expressed itself in angry outbursts toward the nursing staff and a diminishing sense of trust of the medical residents. When I approached Nancy as a result of the nursing staff request, she asked, "You are not going to leave too, are you?" I contracted with Nancy to see her at least once a week or more, if she desired.

As my relationship with Nancy grew, it became apparent that her husband, who was out of work and taking care of three small children, was also in need of someone whom he could talk to. Frank and I would meet in my office on a weekly basis. He used this time to express his feelings of anger, guilt, and depression. Nancy and her husband were under a great deal of stress at this time because of a number of factors. To begin with, it was becoming more and more apparent that Nancy's kidney was rejecting and her course of rejection was longer than that of most patients. Secondly, Nancy's husband and children were forced to live with Nancy's parents during her hospitalization. This was a less than desirable situation. Thirdly, Nancy and her husband were forced to cope with the reality that she soon would be faced with permanent dialysis. This would mean a drastic change in life style for Nancy and her husband since prior to her surgery they had both worked full time and owned their own home. Now Nancy would no longer be able to work and they were considering selling their home. During this period of time, which was approximately 12 weeks, my role with Nancy and her husband was different from the stereotyped role of the pastor or chaplain who is often seen as one who provides the sacraments, offers prayer, or discusses "religious" problems, or the problems of illness in "religious" terms, or the problems of illness in religious language. Rather, my role was that of a person who was available to Nancy and her husband in order that they might have someone within the hospital community to whom they could verbalize their feelings, and ventilate their frustrations. It is interesting to note that Nancy and her husband were Roman Catholic and I am a United Methodist Minister. They were both aware of the fact that I was a chaplain of a different faith, yet this did not seem to interfere with our relationship.

As a member of the renal team, I would act as a one-way intermediary between Nancy and her husband, and the other members of the team, primarily attempting to facilitate communication and understanding. The primary direction of the communication was from Nancy and her husband to the members of the team and the nursing staff on the patient's floor. I attempted to interpret for the staff what I experienced as the focus of Nancy and her husband's emotional stress. During our visits, I also used our time together to help Nancy and her husband clarify the information that they were given by the members of the team and encouraged them to ask questions if they felt unclear.

About the time that Nancy was discharged from the hospital, I began a study leave. Nancy continued to come to the hospital for her dialysis on an outpatient basis. Both Nancy and her husband expressed the desire for continued emotional support; thus I offered to refer Nancy and her husband to our social work staff. Nancy began to see the renal social worker and her husband began to see the social worker assigned to the floor on which Nancy had previously been a patient. (This referral turned out to be quite successful.)

The second patient is Judy, a 24-year-old juvenile diabetic with a complex medical history. She has been totally blind for the past two years and has experienced cardiac stress which, I am told, is related to her diabetes and kidney failure. Her husband Bob is a local clergyman and I have known both Judy and Bob for the past two years. I have followed Judy through many hospitalizations; in each case Judy felt that her medical condition was worsening. Although a kidney transplant had been planned for over a year, Judy's kidneys continued to function and thus dialysis was not required until a week or so before her transplant. Judy's donor was her mother.

During Judy's hospitalizations, she was characterized by many of the hospital staff as "the ideal patient." She rarely complained about her care and showed little upset or frustration with her illness. Although Judy was occasionally seen crying by the nursing staff, there seemed to be a general feeling that she was coping as well as could be expected. I experienced Judy as a person who felt a need to retain self-control. This need for control may be partially explained by the fact that Judy is the wife of a parish minister. The external, as well as internal role expectation which she adhered to was that a good Christian, especially if she is the minister's wife, should be able to steer a fairly stable course emotionally. "Negative" feelings such as anger, fear of dying, hopelessness, etc., are thus not acceptable. Although Judy rarely expressed these feelings, it became evident during our visits that they were there. The first few experiences of dialysis seemed to be more than Judy could cope with, and she began to express at length her anger and frustration and her guilt for having these feelings.

The focus of my relationship with Judy was as "God's representative" to allow her the opportunity to ventilate her feelings and to help her, through our ongoing relationship, to realize that these feelings were both normal and acceptable to God. Thus, "faith language and resources" were explicitly used at different points throughout our relationship.

Like Nancy, Judy also needed to have a consistent relationship with one person throughout her many hospitalizations. It was felt by the Renal Committee that since I had known Judy for the longest period of time, and since religious faith was an important resource for her, I should be the primary staff source of emotional support. Judy reinforced this perception by deciding to limit her lengthy discussion about her feelings to her husband and me. I would communiate what I felt would be helpful for her by writing in Judy's chart and discussing her case during our weekly rounds. During her last admission, Judy went through a stage of withdrawal immediately after her kidney transplant. During this time I used the "psyche" rounds session of the renal committee as an opportunity to consult with the psychiatrist and renal social worker, as well as other members of the renal team, in order to gain insight into the meaning of this withdrawal and the form that our interaction with Judy should take. Later that evening the psychiatrist, Judy's surgeon and nephrologist, and I visited Judy to clinically evaluate her withdrawal.

The weekend before her transplant surgery Judy asked to see me. Judy stated that she felt a need to discuss with me what type of funeral service she would like to have, "just in case I die." Although Judy denied any fear of death, she sensed a felt need to discuss the possibility of her death which she felt might occur either during her surgery or soon thereafter. She began this discussion by asking that I conduct her funeral service, then proceeded to outline the content of such a service. We used this opportunity to also discuss what life had meant for her in the past and what she looked forward to in the future. The following day, Judy and her husband met with me in my office to continue our discussion and record in writing plans for both of their funeral services. Judy and her husband exhibited a style of coping in which there seemed to be a lack of appropriate denial. At the same time it was my perception that they were both exhibiting anticipatory grief reactions. For in a real sense Judy would be a different person after her transplant surgery, regardless of whether the transplant was a success or a failure. If the transplant succeeded, then it would mean a new and more enjoyable life-style for both Bob and Judy. If the kidney rejected, then Judy and Bob would be forced to face life-long dialysis, which would be a new and difficult experience for both of them. But regardless of what transpired, Judy would never be the same person she had been prior to her surgery.

The third and final patient I would like to discuss is John, who was referred to me by a staff nurse working on the floor where he was a patient. Like the other two patients, John was a juvenile onset diabetic. He was 31 years old, blind, and suffering from many medical complications which had begun a year and a half before, soon after the rejection of a kidney he had received from a cadaver donor. John was separated from his wife and living with his parents.

When I met John, about a year and a half ago, he was beginning to go blind and was experiencing a great deal of hand pain, related to a lack of circulation to the middle fingers on both hands. John was a very bright young man who had a Master's Degree in Philosophy and at the age of 31 was a university librarian. John was well liked by the medical and nursing staff who cared for him, apparently because of his strong will to live, his open and active mind, and his age, which was similar to many of the other staff members. John's philosophical background was evident in our relationship. Religion was something to explore and discuss on an intellectual level. But as John grew more ill over the year and a half that I knew him, religious faith became more of a personal struggle.

Kidney failure and blindness caused John to make an abrupt change in his lifestyle. His marriage ended. He had to give up his job. He once again became dependent upon his parents. (Thus, he was treated once again like a young boy.) John had many admissions into the hospital over this year and a half and much of the time that I spent with him was in silence. John had a difficult time expressing his feelings, especially of anger about his illness and the loss of control over his life. It seemed as though his ability to decide when and to whom he would talk was one of the only ways he still was able to exhibit a sense control. Thus, much of my ministry to John was through my presence alone. Often after a silent visit John would thank me for coming and ask me to return soon. During John's stay at the hospital, I spent a great deal of time with his parents, who visited daily, and with the nurses who cared for John.

John's parents drive approximately 80 miles round trip each day to see their son. And if they were unable to visit, they were very apologetic about their absence. This led me to believe that they were experiencing a deep sense of guilt about John's illness, as though they had to make up for some failure on their own part as parents. I felt that it was important to give them a great deal of emotional support; they were hurting over the slow death of their son and they needed a shoulder to cry on. I also attempted to convey to them through my role as chaplain, that in God's eyes, they had not failed. If they wanted to be with John that was okay, but it was also okay to take a day off to get some rest. I also attempted to aid John's parents in doing their anticipatory grief work by allowing and encouraging them to talk about John as he used to be before his illness. Beyond its benefits to John's parents, this discussion also helped me to gain a holistic picture of who John was as a person. And finally, I attempted to provide support and a sense of God's presence as John's family decided how or what to tell him when it became apparent the dialysis was no longer medically possible.

Many of the medical staff who cared for John—floor nurses, dialysis unit nurses, and doctors—found that it was emotionally draining to care for this man. At one time or another he rendered each of us helpless. This brought feelings of frustration, anger, grief, and guilt. During these times, I would attempt to minister to the staff by encouraging them to ventilate their feelings and to share openly and honestly my own pain. When it became apparent that dialysis was no longer possible, I not only spent time with John's family but I also attempted to minister to the attending physician and the nursing staff who had cared for John during his last admission. Those who come to know a patient in a very caring and intimate way over a long period of time also need to be ministered to when the patient dies, for they too experience grief and loss. The renal social worker and I had come to know and care deeply for John and his family. After John's death we attended his funeral and a church-sponsored meal after the funeral, at which time we sat with John's family. This was a way for us to grieve over the loss which we had experienced. For John's family our presence seemed to symbolize that the hospital was more than an institution; it was people who really cared about their son and about them.

For those of us who care for renal patients and especially for those renal patients who are also diabetics, there is often a sense that we are involved in the care of terminally ill patients. In such circumstances despair and hopelessness at times haunt patients, family, and staff alike. In religious tradition the clergy has historically been called the doctor of the soul. It has been my purpose in this chapter to show that the presence of the chaplain on the hemodialysis and kidney transplant team can, through his ministry, offer hope in the midst of despair, and can further enhance the healing of the body through the healing of the spirit. But if renewed health becomes unrealistic, as was the case with John, the chaplain can "be" with the patient and those who care for him. In the midst of their fear and loss, he stands as a reminder that death, though it remains a mystery, is yet a part of life, and in the sight of God we remain acceptable, cared for, and loved.

ACKNOWLEDGMENT. In conclusion, I would like to thank my fellow members of the Department of Pastoral Care and the members of the renal team for their knowledge and help in making this chapter possible, and Dr. Norman Levy, who as editor of this book has graciously given me the opportunity to share this work.

REFERENCES

1. JOHNSON, PAUL E. *Psychology of pastoral care.* New York, Nashville: Abingdon Press, 1953, p. 24.
2. CAREY, RAYMOND G. *Hospital chaplains: who needs them?* St. Louis: The Catholic Hospital Association, 1972, p. 86.
3. JOHNSON, A. WAYLAND, and GUNNING, KEVIN. Reflections on kidney transplantation and renal dialysis. *Bulletin of the American Protestant Hospital Association,* 1977, XLI, 96.
4. PRUYSER, PAUL W. *The minister as diagnostician.* Philadelphia: The Westminster Press, 1976, pp. 10, 60.

8

The Nephrology Social Worker as the Primary Psychological Practitioner

JOSEPH G. TRAMO

In perusing the literature of psychosocial factors associated with end-stage renal disease, it is not unusual to find frequent references to inter-disciplinary cooperation and team interaction. The reason for this is rather simple, for, in the relatively few years of dialysis/transplant development, it has become more and more apparent that the support systems surrounding this particular patient group are unique in concept and function. In no other area of medical specialty is the concentration of staff–patient contact as intense or ongoing, so intimately related to treatment and success or failure of this treatment. One finds it hard to compare even the myriad of cancer therapies or the strenuous mechanics of rehabilitation medicine to the crowded scale of day to day, medical and social attention that is rained upon the patient held captive by his kidney failure. Working in this arena, a professional feels the impact of loss and dependency more strongly than in other specialty areas and hears more clearly the call for psychological support from these patients who are neither well nor dying, fully dependent nor free, and neither in control nor fully without it.

The above portrait of ambivalence, the dilemma of the dialysis patient, poses a challenge to the staff who meet this patient routinely. There has never been a question in determining who balances the purely medical matters in a unit, but a minor battle still rages as to who can masterfully manage the psychological and social upheavals that are distinctly present. Who among nurse, technician, dietician, psychologist, social worker, or psychiatrist is to handle these situations: One or everyone? If

JOSEPH G. TRAMO, M.S.S.S., A.C.S.W. • Chief Social Worker, Division of Medical Social Services, Temple University Hospital; Field Instructor, Temple University School of Social Administration, Philadelphia, Pennsylvania.

the treatment of psychosocial conflict is not a special task, then any staff member can do it. I believe, however, that this is not true, and the patient should not be the victim of a territorial war, as each well intentioned staff person tries to secure the title of ultimate psychosocial therapist of the unit. It is chaotic, this tug-of-war, and detrimental to patient care and team work alike.

A key to the resolution of this conflict lies in a belief that each discipline in an end-stage renal disease unit has a primary task. Blending of purpose will occur in nonmedical areas and is impossible to prevent. But if some definitive sense of professional responsibility and expertise cannot be agreed upon, then we can only continue to flounder in a pool of partial talents and inefficiency.

Presumption should not be read into the statement that the nephrology social worker is the primary psychological practitioner; it is not meant to be a challenge. Most professionals working on a dialysis/transplant team will, at some time or other, be drawn more deeply into a patient's social and emotional problems than they are prepared to handle. Do they attempt to deal with the problem and the ramifications which will most certainly follow? Are they trained specifically to do this or do they refer the situation to someone whose education has prepared and mandated him to work with various kinds of personal relationships?

The nephrology social worker is a professional, trained over an intensive two-year period in the principles of human growth and behavior and the skills needed to work purposefully with people toward regaining their equilibrium when it is out of synchronization with the psychosocial milieu. It is a course of study which introduces and strengthens knowledge of adaptive and defensive mechanisms so that helping persons in conflict becomes more than simply using logic or common sense to arrive at solutions. It is an attempt, as well, at individual examination of personal patterns of behavior so that the social worker can more easily be master of his own frustration to profit the handicapped person, thereby learning that he cannot answer anxiety with anxiety without blocking the process of change.

By definition of function, the social worker uses himself through the development of a sensitive relationship with a person in trouble and through manipulation and mobilization of environmental resources, to help that person to recognize his own abilities to lessen, adapt to, or end conflict. The end result is that this person may regain some degree of harmony within his social and psychological environment. The social work profession is governed by values which respect individual rights and differences and a belief in the individual's basic dignity. It is this body of knowledge and code of ethics, which sanctions the social worker to work with people toward change.

As suggested earlier on in this chapter, the person being treated in a dialysis/transplant unit can easily be seen as standing alone among people in any other chronic disease group. Here is a fusion of psychological and social problems which is of a degree that surpasses similarities to the others. In few other forms of chronic illness does one have to cope with so much so simultaneously. There is the presence of the machine which imposes dependency yet, unlike the other machine dominated illnesses, proffers independence in an almost teasing way. A special diet and numerous medications keep the kidney patient in constant awareness of his fragility. Omnipresent is the staff of professionals always in watch, monitoring the routine and boredom of the schedule. There are sometimes sudden changes in sexual response, and the always distressing possible loss of job security; loss of control, and the discovery that this loss can paradoxically lead to use of new controls over life and other people's lives. Add to all this the severe limitations and demands on a family, and it is obvious that the changes are catastrophic, affecting many people and the individual's living space dramatically.

As a patient with kidney failure is initiated into the renal disease system, it is essential that consideration be given to the unique mixture of emotional and social upheaveal that suddenly arises out of the medical situation and tends to overpower the patient and the people important to him. An adequately descriptive psychosocial evaluation should be started early in the patient's awareness of what is in the future in regards to his illness. This core of information will allow for some prediction, through understanding of individual and family coping competencies, as to how any patient will react to the impending strenuous regimen. Such preliminary data are invaluable to staff and patient alike in helping unravel the tangled messages and rules that lead to dissatisfaction, disenchantment, and dysfunction once treatment begins.

The nephrology social worker is the professional in a unit prepared to assemble and analyze the total picture of such patients, particularly any whose social experience is completely upturned by all that chronic kidney failure involves. In most dialysis units, the social worker is the only person with expertise in using the interview as both a mechanism for gathering pertinent data and as a treatment form. It is this person who is most likely seen by the family and the patient as concerned primarily with the nonmedical details of a frightening, complicating illness. And it is through the initial evaluations that the first shocks of change are ventilated and scrutinzied with the patient in terms of seeking solutions.

It is of greatest importance that the fears generated in the beginning stages of a person's introduction to dialysis be recognized and approached without hesitation. Certainly a great part of any patient's maladaptation to dialysis is a result of vague preparation for the intricacies of the treatment. More often than not, no opportunity is given to meet the anxieties squarely and to discuss all possible alternatives in order to successfully manage the changes that will occur.

It is the nephrology social worker's responsibility to be available at this crucial time, ready to meet with the family, to connect with the community, and to interpret meaning and convey unresolved concerns directly from patient to primary physician. The future of any supportive relationship depends highly on the success of communication during these initial contacts. From this relationship ideally come the facts on which are based the treatment plans best suited to each patient's individual style of adaption. From the start of the evaluation, through the transition period, and on into full realization of the permanence of treatment, the trained social worker is the person most available to both patient and family in assisting them to handle the psychosocial fallout. This is the team member who will most aptly be following through with nonmedical issues by right of training and, most importantly, by area of responsibility to the patient–family–community group.

A key factor in this vital area of patient care is the assumption that the social worker on the nephrology team has duties exclusive to that service. Only in this way can the helping relationship have a firm beginning, since the patient can be approached as an out-patient, followed as an inpatient, and then brought less threateningly into the unit. This gradual buildup of support is particularly important when transplant is feasible. The social worker will begin counselling at the earliest stages of discussion, evaluating family, and helping the patient examine the fears and ambivalences of organ transplant. By the time the patient reaches the dialysis machine, many emotions have been unraveled so that the pressure of immediate decisions can be avoided.

Emotional and psychological crises can occur at any time along the continuum from the commencement of dialysis and, certainly, once it has become a fully instituted treatment. The imposition of a dialysis regimen on a person can create enough stress so that problems coped with previously seem insurmountable additions to an already overloaded emotional circuit. Intervening in the crises, the social worker makes use of the detailed file of social and psychological data in attempting to assist the patient in looking for resolutions to the problems. This entails a skillful analysis of the data so that a patient is not simply consoled by an aphorism and a sympathetic pat on the back.

In three brief examples, the kinds of problems encountered and the social worker's action in relation to them may help pinpoint the particular role of this professional in the team. It is essential to note in the examples how the social agitation and concomitant emotional disharmony are attended to simultaneously to effect a return to some semblance of past psychosocial order. It is in this welding of two components of human interaction that the most unique aspect of social work can be identified. Certainly, for patients embroiled in the anxieties of a chronic kidney disease program, this skill for reestablishing balance, through application of various social and psychosocial principles, is a service which must necessarily be provided.

A 24-year-old woman's kidney function ceased at a time in her life when she was just beginning to pull her life together. For two years her 3-year-old son had been in foster care, put there by a variety of circumstances that were as complex as the means to overcome them. She was, however, close to succeeding, for she had been trying determinedly to become vocationally and financially secure enough to have her boy returned to her home. Suddenly, kidney disease put her out of work and almost out of her mind, until she became immobile and depressed.

The unit social worker spent up to an hour at a time with the patient whenever she was on treatment. The shared communications of these one-to-one sessions helped her ventilate her anger at the reversals caused by her illness. The social worker examined with her all the by-products of the disease and how, in reality, they had limited her progress. They discussed many alternatives that might lead to new pathways to her former goals, but only after the social worker helped her understand the naturalness of her depression and resultant disconcerting loss of interest in her children. She needed to feel less guilty and less personally responsible for the sense of having crushed the hopes of her family. Later, by employing community resources and concentrating on the most appropriate of a limited number of vocational guidance aids, he successfully helped her find employment again.

A sizable portion of effort in this situation was devoted to the social worker's advocacy on behalf of the patient with a sceptical foster home agency. Many contacts with the agency's staff were made to dispel the misinterpretations of the patient's lack of energy as signs of abandonment. Considerable time was spent in carrying out this prime social work role, so that proceedings aimed at claiming the patient an unfit mother would be stopped. By the end of her first year on dialysis, the child was taken out of care.

In a second situation, the social worker became involved in helping a 60-year-old woman overcome an overwhelming grief reaction. Only a few weeks after she had begun a chronic dialysis schedule, her closest brother died from a pulmonary embolism. Her normally strong ego was paralyzed, and no amount of well intentioned concern from the staff was conducive to her regrouping her defenses. Finally, when the staff subjectively decided that her grieving period was extending beyond what they felt should be its limit, they became impatient with her. Her sudden weeping spells and overall moroseness made her a virtual pariah among some of the staff, and her noncompliance visibly irritated them.

Since the social worker knew a lot about this patient's family relationships through a thorough predialysis psychosocial evaluation, they were brought into the process of treatment through frequent phone contacts and, when able, by making visits to the unit. The strong family bonds proved to be vastly supportive and were employed by the social worker to shore up the patient's weakened defenses. After four months of casework on an almost daily basis, she began to regain control. The staff discussed the progress of the change in patient care conferences and their understanding helped restore concord in the unit.

Finally, a 55-year-old man had been a frustrating source of dialysis unit chaos because of his manipulative behavior. A former boxer and still a heavy abuser of alcohol, he was becoming more painfully aware with every dialysis that his masculine identity and sexual prowess had also been destroyed along with his kidney's capacity to function. He tried to compensate for his losses by controlling every situation he could that connected to the limitations of his disease. He played at being passive with the nursing staff. He would trap them into making decisions for him, then attempt to make them feel guilty if they hurt him by making what he claimed was the wrong decision. He engaged the technicians and nurses in battle by subtly pitting one's concern for him against the others'. He was maddening and unrelenting!

The social worker was most identifiably available to concentrate on the man's shattered self-respect. This was demonstrated by the development of a relationship solely directed to what was most important to that patient in that space of time. And what was paramount was not his medical status or his nursing care or the techniques of his dialysis, but the means he was going to need to regain his sense of being a complete and worthwhile person. By skillful use of a guileless one-to-one interaction, a foundation was laid for constructive cooperation. The control issue came into sharper focus when the patient saw it as his way of neutralizing the frightening loss of self-esteem. Then the social worker singled out staff members who were particularly stressed by the patient's behavior. Through informal discussions and broader studies during full team conferences, the underlying reasons for the patient's disruptiveness were analyzed. The team was requested, as well, to examine their own dread in trying to cope with the obvious threats to their integrity which occurred whenever the patient provoked them into submitting to his demands.

During this delving into inner personality factors with patient and staff, the social worker was also probing the community in which the patient lived to discover what resources were usable in helping him establish a sense of stability. This was actualized by reacquainting him with an athletic club in the neighborhood and helping him secure a part-time job in a gym. The manipulative gestures lessened and, though he relapsed into phases of uncooperativeness during recurrent physical crises, he was quicker to appreciate the staff's reciprocal anger.

In these cases, the nephrology social worker was the member of the renal team to whom the problems were referred and who worked directly with each patient toward resolution of the conflict. In each instance, there was consultation with the physician and nursing staff on the current medical circumstances of the patient. A comprehension of what chemical imbalances and other physical malfunctions exist cannot be separated from the essence of possible causes for behavior changes, depressions, anxieties, and sudden emotional eruptions.

In two of these cases there was also consultation with psychiatrists who were available to the specific units. Their opinions were basically the same, that no psychiatric intervention was necesary and that such intervention might be detrimental to the relationship already established by the social worker. In reality, most dialysis units have very few patients who use the skills of psychiatry when a social worker, with a firm academic and experiential background in psychosocial supportive casework, is functioning professionally.

Unquestionably every staff person in a dialysis/transplant setting must be alert to the psychological and social maelstroms that can toss their patients completely off balance. But they should also be aware of how best to go about the job of restoring that balance. To avoid the consternation that comes with duplication of service and competition, there must be recognition that each discipline has its primary task. Blending which does occur, therefore, is a shared work experience rather than a battle for supremacy. While it is unacceptable to define "primary" as most important or only, in the context of the interaction with patients by all professionals in a unit, the nephrology social worker, in the facilities of most renal disease programs, is the first available and most continuous psychological practitioner with patients and families. In this sense, and in light of what I have illustrated here, this professional is the primary psychological practitioner.

SELECTED BIBLIOGRAPHY

ABRAM, H. S. The psychiatrist, the treatment of chronic renal failure, and the prolongation of life: II. *American Journal of Psychiatry*, 1969, 126, 157–166.
BUCHANAN, D.C., and ABRAM, H. S. Psychological adaptation to chronic hemodialysis. *Dialysis and Transplantation*, 1976, 5(2), 36–42, 84.
GOLDMEIER, J. The social worker. *Dialysis and Transplantation*, 1973, 2(3), 10.
HICKEY, K. Impact of kidney disease on patient, family, and society. *Social Casework*, 1972, 53(7), 391–398.
KAPLAN DE-NOUR, A., CZACZKES, J. W., and LELOS, P. A study of chronic hemodialysis teams—differences in opinions and expectations. *Journal of Chronic Diseases*, 1972, 25, 441–448.
LANDSMAN, M. The renal social worker in a sattelite. *Dialysis and Transplantation*, 1976, 5(3), 25–26.
LOWE, J. I., and HERRANEN, M. Conflict in teamwork: Understanding roles and relationships. *Social Work in Health Care*, 1978, 3(3), 323–330.
MACNAMARA, M. Psychosocial problems in a renal unit. *British Journal of Psychiatry*, 1967, 113, 1231–1236.
MAILICK, M. D., and JORDON, P. A multimodel approach to collaborative practice in health settings. *Social Work in Health Care*, 1977, 2(4), 445–453.
NATIONAL ASSOCIATION OF SOCIAL WORKERS. *Code of Ethics* (Amended ed.). April, 1967.

78 JOSEPH G. TRAMO

PERLMAN, H. H. *Social casework: a problem solving process*. Chicago: University of Chicago Press, 1957.

RICHMOND, M. E. *Social diagnosis* (Paperback ed.). New York: Free Press, 1965.

SHORT, M. J. Roles of denial in chronic hemodialysis. *Archives of General Psychiatry*, 1969, 20, 433–437.

WALSER, D. Behavioral effects of dialysis. *The Canadian Nurse*, 1974, 70, 23–25.

9
A Family-Oriented Supportive Approach to Dialysis and Renal Transplantation in Children

Dennis Drotar, Mary Ann Ganofsky, Sudesh Makker, and Denise DeMaio

Introduction

Comprehensive pediatric care provided by an interdisciplinary team is often recommended to help families cope with the considerable stresses involved in dialysis and renal transplantation.[1] The various functions of comprehensive care include emotional support of families through the course of treatment, attention to the child's psychosocial adjustment, and facilitation of patient–physician communications. The structure and emphasis of comprehensive care program vary considerably from setting to setting. This report describes the role of one comprehensive care team in aiding family coping and helping families with treatment decisions, with particular reference to renal transplantation.

The Setting and Structure of Comprehensive Care

The pediatric nephrology program of Case Western Reserve University Medical School and Rainbow Babies and Childrens Hospital serves as the major referral center in Northeastern Ohio for children with end-stage renal failure. Since 1972, the team has supervised a total of 26 transplants. Our relatively small program has allowed us to have intensive contact with children and their families. Care is supervised by a core team from

Dennis Drotar, Ph.D. • Associate Professor in Pediatrics and Psychiatry; Mary Ann Ganofsky, A.C.S.W. • Staff Social Worker; Sudesh Makker, M.D. • Associate Professor of Pediatrics; Denise DeMaio, R.N., M.A., • Pediatric Nephrology, Case Western Reserve Medical School; and Rainbow Babies and Childrens Hospital, Cleveland, Ohio.

pediatric nephrology including three full time pediatric faculty, two renal fellows, a full time pediatric nurse clinician, nurses and technicians from the dialysis unit, and staff and trainees from social work, dietary, and psychology.

Initially, the pediatric staff had sole responsibility for communications with and support of families. However, our experience with children and families whose severe adjustment problem warranted intensive psychosocial intervention indicated the need for a broader, interdisciplinary approach. Since end stage renal failure presents stresses to all families, it seemed judicious to develop a program to support all families, not just the severely disturbed, through their arduous journey through the course of treatment.[2,3] Our experience suggested the quality of the individual child's adjustment depends to a large extent on the families' coping skills, particularly their ability to communicate concerning the child's illness. Thus, our program gradually evolved to emphasize emotional decisions. The provision of information and support to families at critical junctures of treatment, such as the onset of renal disease, is an important feature of this family oriented model of care. Discussions with the entire family, parents and family subgroups, supplement the work with the child. For example, once it is apparent that the child will go into renal failure, the parents, the child, and other family members participate in a meeting which is also attended by the pediatric nephrologist, social worker, and nurse clinician. Family members listen to a discussion of the nature of chronic renal failure, the physiology, complications, and treatment. From the outset, family members are given ample opportunity to express their reactions to the child's physical status and treatment. In addition, other family members' reactions to the affected child's condition and treatment are also solicited.

However, these discussions are not restricted to the child's medical problems. From the outset, we feel it is important to review the child's adaptation to life tasks, such as school. In this way, we reinforce the importance of the families' attention to the child's overall psychosocial adjustment. In the heat of difficult decisions raised by the child's overall psychosocial adjustment, one can easily lose sight of the child's adjustment to life tasks. We find that repetition of our instructions to the family is especially important. Thus, while the child is on dialysis, periodic family meetings are held to review the child's treatment and family's adaptation.

The presentation of information concerning transplantation to families has presented a continuing dilemma to the treatment team. Realizing that both the treatment team and the family are locked into a treatment course that they have not chosen, we have tried to enhance the families' sense of control and unity by helping them to weigh treatment alternatives as a group. The family is given detailed information concerning the benefits and hazards of transplantation. We do not tell families that they must go through with transplantation. Instead, the family is asked to discuss the alternatives as a group and engage in dialogue with the treatment team. We try to slow the normally rapid course of family decision making concerning transplantation by having a number of sit down discussions with the families involving such questions as whether to proceed with transplant, the timing of transplant, and the choice of donor. Once a decision for transplant has been reached, the team tries to be continually available to family members to help them ventilate feelings and answer questions. A good deal of time is devoted to prepare the donor and recipient for the concrete details of the hospitalization such as the specific tests, procedures, and the discomfort involved. We find that donors begin to work through their worries almost immediately. For example, our sibling and parent donors have been concerned that they might get kidney disease, that their life-style might be changed or that they may be hurt by the surgery or anesthesia. When given an opportunity, some donors discuss their concerns about the decision itself, particularly their feelings of constraint, as articulated nicely by a 18-year-old sibling donor: "They told us we had a near-perfect match. When they tell you that there isn't much choice. The bottom line is you don't have much choice."

At the time of transplant, the team tries to insure support for the donor as well as the recipient. Donors have expressed their appreciation for this support. For example, one father commented: "It all happened so fast, it was scary. I was scared all the way to the operating room . . . but all the extra attention helped keep my mind off the worries." A mother stated: "They (the team) came in often and looked at us . . . it let you know that you are still a part of this. It was not 'we are done with you lady.' "

In the crisis period following transplant, the team enhances family coping by providing reassurance, repetition of information concerning procedures, and clarification of communications. To help further family support, parent or sibling donors room together with the recipient. This approach was an outgrowth of our clinical experiences with Phil, and his mother who donated his kidney. The transplant had been a grueling experience for the whole family. Immediately following transplant, we had particular concern about the mother's adjustment. Although we were not responsible for the mother's care, we visited her and brought progress reports of Phil. However, she seemed quite depressed and had many somatic complaints, despite the fact that the postsurgical course for both mother and son was going reasonably well. Phil was also somewhat depressed. We noted that when mother visited Phil, he was brighter, more alert, and more involved in his own care. She also seemed to benefit from the visits. This suggested to us that mother and child would prosper if they had direct and steady access to each other throughout the recuperative process. The staff on the young adult unit who had prior experience with adult patients agreed to accept the mother from the adult surgical division. Phil and his mother's affect brightened considerably following this move. The mother involved herself in Phil's care and became more active. The family pulled together to weather the storm of a mild rejection episode, and the remainder of the hospitalization went well. The mother was discharged after about a week. However, she and other family members continued to visit Phil. We felt that this procedure lessened everyone's anxiety and facilitated the treatment team's communications to the family.

We have now tried this approach with a number of donors and recipients and have interviewed them concerning their reactions. Generally, the donors have appreciated the support and lack of restrictions of being on the unit. All of the donors reported the advantage of knowing the recipient's condition, and the resultant feeling of security. For example, one mother said that the major advantage was "knowing what was going on all the time. If I was in another place, I would have been going crazy, not knowing." Many donors and recipients have also indicated that this approach aided family closeness. For example, a girl responded to the question "What was it like to have your mother in the same room as you?" with: "Loving, because I was with someone I loved." One father noted: "It was a damned good idea to be in the same room, a good feeling to look at him asleep and know I'd given him a kidney." At the same time, some of the donors articulated the problems posed by the close contact. For example, one father said that he had some anxious moments when his son felt pains, "It's hard to see your son hurting." Another mother stated: "She was feeling a lot better than I was, she wanted to walk around, wanted me to come to her bed, but I resented this, because she wanted me to comfort her when I felt so bad." Nursing support of the child is critical because it is most certainly unfair to ask the parents to assume this responsibility. One 13-year-old recipient expressed annoyance because his father was "over-protective": "Anything they did to me, he'd have to know about it." To discourage undue closeness among donor and recipient and permit the donor's expression of anger, opportunities are provided for donor and recipient to express the feelings individually. In addition, we have taken pains to help the parents recognize and deal with the excessive dependency that can flower in the posttransplant period.

During the hospitalization for the transplant, the social worker and nurse clinician visit with the family frequently, seven days a week, two or three times a day. These visits supplement the physician's communications and help the family ventilate the inevitable frustration that surround transplantation. If the parents have a concern and their physican is not available, the social worker will track this information down for the parents. This is particularly important in view of the inevitable departures from the planned pattern of care which can occur in the posttransplant period. As soon as the child can go home, yet another meeting is arranged with the family to go over the care of the transplant. In this meeting, the team discusses the transplant, the problem of rejection, diet, and drugs. We feel it is important to prepare the child and family for the massive changes in routine and body image which occur soon after transplant and can be avoided in the euphoria which surrounds a successful transplant. Based on our knowledge of the family, we anticipate possible problem areas, emphasizing the importance of patient compliance with diet, particularly medication. We repeatedly stress the danger of kidney rejection and strongly discourage the child's experimenting with the medication. The transition from the child's being "sick" with renal failure to being "well" with the transplant can be a difficult one. For this reason, strong emphasis is placed on the child's return to daily routine and responsibilities. Regression in the child's functioning can occur following transplantation particularly if the parents continue to view the child as overly vulnerable or sick. Some parents may try to make things up to their child by not placing any demands on them, a pattern which can result in school avoidance and isolation from peers. The team takes an active, parentlike stance in making plans for the child's return to school before discharge. If the child and parents were overly close prior to the transplant, chances are that this closeness may be intensified following transplantation. Such problems are discussed in the family meetings. Immediately following transplantation, the patients and their families are followed closely, initially once a week and then less often, depending on the child's physical status. Consistent with the experience of others[4] we often encounter "let downs" in the posttransplant period as the parents and patients come to terms with the chronicity of their condition and their altered physical appearance. The team tries to give permission for the child to get angry at the medication that makes them fat and at peers who tease them. At the same time, the need for the child and family to adhere to the treatment regimen is reemphasized. During this time, one can uncover the child's misperceptions of explanations, which may not have been accurately understood because of anxiety. For example, one 11-year-old girl expressed surprise to our nurse clinician when the reason for the prednisone medication was again explained to her. She said, "Why, I thought it was helping me grow."

ENHANCING FAMILY PARTICIPATION IN DECISION MAKING

The management of end-stage renal failure places great stress on the physician–family relationship.[5] Families' expectations for the physician to cure the illness are not met. Instead, the parents are asked to assume a difficult treatment regimen which requires compliance with diet and medication, the intrusion of dialysis, and living with the fears of kidney rejection. In our experience, families' ambivalence about this burdensome treatment regimen may have a number of maladaptive consequences. Some parents withdraw their energies from the child who is expected to cope with "his" problem independently. Over time, some families make themselves unavailable to the treatment staff, to avoid confronting difficult decisions. Our experience suggests the need for a continuing dialogue between the treatment team and families concerning the child's treatment.

Decisions involving dialysis vs. transplant, the timing of transplantation, live related donors vs. cadaver kidney, and the choice of donor are often difficult. The relative advantages and disadvantages of each alternative must be weighed with reference to the child's physical status, safety, quality of life, and the stresses on the family. For this reason, we try to balance the responsibility for decision making between the team and family by securing family members' opinions and listening to their reactions. This approach has a number of advantages: First, it allows families to express their fears and to anticipate feelings that may arise later. Families often need permission to express their ambivalence about the treatments that are keeping their child alive. Families' discussion of treatment alternatives helps prepare them for the changes in family routines required by the treatments. Families can negotiate these shifts in treatment more adaptively if they feel like they are participants in rather than passive recipients of treatment.

The potential role of the treatment team in helping families with the decision for transplantation is illustrated in the case of Jeannie, a 7-year-old girl, who is the youngest in a family of eight.

> The parents were previously married and Jeannie has a very valued position in this family as the only child of this union. Her problems included chronic renal failure, small stature (she is about the size of a 3- to 4-year-old), and mild mental retardation. The family was from a small community an hour and a half away from the center and enjoyed the support of many people within the community. The maternal grandparents were very active caretakers for Jeannie. In addition, the family's affiliation with their church and their involvement with their pastor also were important supports for them.
>
> When we first saw Jeannie and her family, Jeannie was the youngest and smallest child to be considered for hemodialysis in our program. The various treatment options were discussed including constraints of dialyzing a small

child. The family requested to discuss Jeannie with us and their pastor, who had had some experience with dialysis patients in his ministry. The mother, Mrs. S., tearfully asked whether she should submit Jeannie to the discomforts of dialysis with all its uncertainties. She was understandably concerned with the demands that would be placed on her family. Unable to discuss these issues with her husband, Mrs. S. was concerned that something bad might happen to him if anything happened to Jeannie. Mrs. S. shared her feelings with her physician, social worker, and pastor and gradually became more convined that dialysis was "right" for Jeannie. Nevertheless, she still felt trapped in this difficult decision. Jeannie began dialysis with her parents' shaky acceptance but she had difficulties: She was quite active and did not like to lie still in bed. Frequently demanding to sit up in bed, she occasionally hit staff when annoyed or upset. Knowing the parents' feelings of responsibility for Jeannie, we were available to discuss her adjustment to dialysis with them. Fortunately, Jeannie's behavioral problems on dialysis did not extend to her behavior in school, with peers, or with family. During the next five months, we did not have much contact with Mrs. S. because other family members brought Jeannie to dialysis. However, Mr. S. became increasingly concerned about his wife's anxiety. Since the parents could not express their worries to one another, we arranged for a joint discussion with them. During this meeting, we reviewed Jeannie's medical and psychosocial progress, including her delayed development which had recently been evaluated. We discussed expectations for Jeannie's future, that she would continue to make developmental progress, but at a slower than normal rate. We also raised the question of transplantation at this meeting. The siblings had expressed concern that Jeannie would not be self-sufficient and that their mother should not take a chance with her own well being by donating a kidney. On the other hand, the parents did not want Jeannie to continue on hemodialysis, given her problematic adjustment. With our assurance that a transplant was possible (although not without complications) the parents decided to go ahead with surgery. Mrs. S. readily offered herself as a donor. Further support was given to siblings to help them understand and accept the parents' decision. Jeannie had a successful transplantation and has maintained adequate adjustment at home and at school. Her siblings have been very involved with her and Mrs. S. has been able to return to work for the first time in two and a half years. Although Mrs. S. is still concerned about Jeannie's future, particularly about kidney rejection, she and her family have coped well with these uncertainties.

We have also encountered situations where families have great difficulty taking responsibility for treatment related decisions. Parental abdication of responsibility for decision making often reflects their anxiety and proves quite troubling for the staff. In certain instances, it is helpful for the team to take a more active role in making a firm recommendation for treatment that appears in the child's interest.

This dilemma was illustrated in our recent experiences with an 11-year-old girl, Dinah, who had renal failure due to cystinosis. Initially, Dinah, a 10-kg child, was too small to be transplanted. Unfortunately, her treatment course on dialysis was extremely difficult and included many complications such as seizures and infections. Dinah's emotional development also suffered. She had become fearful of dying and quite withdrawn over the course of treatment. The family was initially set against a transplant as they viewed this as a risky precedure. The parents' fear caused them to look to Dinah for a decision. Each time the possibility of transplant was raised, Dinah remained steadfast in her excuses, "No, not now. Can we wait until next year?" Discussions with ourselves and other patients about the wisdom of this decision could not convince her and her parents. Unfortunately, the parents lived at a distance and contacts with the treatment team had become quite sporadic. We felt the family was avoiding us because they did not want to face the decision. The parents, the child, and treatment team were locked into this uncomfortable status quo for a long time. We had many heated discussions about Dinah and her treatment course. The staff expressed reservations such as "I couldn't live with it if we pushed the family to go through with this and she died." Others stated that taking the risk might be preferable to the quality of life she was currently living. We were also quite angry at the parents for opting out on the treatment and not exercising their responsibility and leaving it to us. On retrospect, we should have exercised our responsibility and made a forceful recommendation for transplant. Most recently, our knowledge that Dinah was becoming increasingly miserable on dialysis troubled us greatly. With some ambivalence, we eventually decided to take matters into our own hands and put her on the cadaver list. This decision was accepted by the parents and Dinah who seemed to feel relief that a decision had been reached. Dinah was transplanted just last week.

ENHANCING TEAM FUNCTIONING AND WORKING WITH STAFF REACTIONS

Providing emotional support to families and helping families come to terms with decisions places great demands on the team members. A family oriented approach cannot be implemented without establishing a mechanism for the team members to share information, make decisions, plan interventions with families, and give support to one another. Professional disciplines in a large medical setting often operate in isolation from one another. In the complex, superspecialized world of the modern pediatric hospital, each professional discipline may have access to only a fragment of the total information, which can interfere with communications with families.[6] Mental health consultants need to be familiar with the nature of renal disease and treatments to have empathy for families' struggles and to make accurate judgments concerning the adequacy of their adjustment.[2] At the same time, the physician must consider the child's and the family's total psychosocial adjustment in his encounters with them to avoid a counterproductive emphasis on the technical aspects of the child's condition.

Team members share responsibility for the planning, the timing, and nature of these medical and psychosocial interventions. More than one team member is usually involved in a given family, necessitating careful structuring of their work. Team members often disagree concerning the most effective approach with families. At our weekly comprehensive care meetings, team members argue, question, and share their concerns about working with different families. Although these encounters can be frustrating, the team's functioning and morale appears to be enhanced by a sharing of decision making. At the same time, the team still requires leadership to make difficult decisions where the team is split. Strong pediatric leadership and support has been a critical component of our comprehensive care program.

Team members' reactions to treatment setbacks, agonizing medical decisions, and the child and family's pain and discomfort can affect the team's emotional climate. In group meetings, feelings of helplessness, e.g., "I don't know what to do" concerning patients and their treatment are often expressed. In addition, concern is often expressed about putting the child through difficult procedures and compromising the child's quality of life.

The staff can benefit from formal and informal means of mutual support to help manage their emotional reactions. In our team, weekly interdisciplinary meetings provide some of this support.[7] In the course of planning their work, various staff members spontaneously express their reactions to their work. Venting anger at a frustrating situation or family is quite common. It is harder for staff to express feelings of sadness, which may be communicated by an uneasy group silence. Humorous comments about the tragic or absurd nature of various clinical situations allow the staff to discharge tension. While it is helpful for the team to recognize their reactions to their work, it is impossible for them to dwell on their reactions in the context of heavy patient care demands. For this reason, it is often helpful to discuss the impact of a given treatment situation, e.g., "this has been really hard for us." Pointing out the similarities and differences in family vs staff reactions can facilitate the staff's empathy for families' distress. In tragic situations involving a serious, life threatening treatment setback, the team's support of one another allows them to maintain their contact with parents and children without prematurely withdrawing from them. The following case example illustrates the role of team support in aiding a family through the extraordinary circumstances of their child's tragic conditions.

> John was a nine-year-old boy in renal failure who had been maintained on hemodialysis with good results concerning his physical growth and emotional adjustment. Following John's second transplant (the first one never functioned), John developed rapid, irreversible rejection which could not be curtailed. Shortly after his return to dialysis, for a still undetermined reason, he suffered severe hypertensive encephaolpathy resulting in seizures, cerebral hemorrhage, and coma. Initially some hope existed that John would

awaken. When the neurologists diagnosed irreversible brain damage, that hope ceased and John remained comatose on hemodialysis. Because the parents expected it and alternatives had not been thought through, three times weekly dialysis continued.

Team members argued the various legal, ethical questions posed by John's condition. The consensus slowly developed that cessation of dialysis would be in the family's best interest. However, this had not been shared with the parents and the team could certainly not make a unilateral decision. The physicians and social worker met with the family frequently to discuss John's condition and to answer their questions.

The mother and grandmother were in constant attendance. The social worker visited the mother once and sometimes twice a day, seven days a week. The conversation ranged from superficial topics to intimate sharing of feelings of her anguish over John's condition and the sense of abandonment she felt from her husband's return to work and his infrequent visits. As the weeks wore on, the stresses on family and staff grew. Feelings of anger and helplessness were expressed on both sides. Eventually our visits with the mother and extensive discussions allowed a consensus to emerge. Late one evening as the social worker was preparing to leave, the mother expressed great distress over the idea that John would require a nasal–gastric tube for feeding. Her upset concerned more than just the tube so the social worker and she moved to an empty room. There the mother slowly, but quite articulately talked about everything she had been feeling during the previous weeks. Her feelings paralleled the renal team's. She said that John would not want to live in his unconscious state. She saw only pain being inflicted with no chance of any improvement. Yet, she felt that she could not make the decision to stop dialysis by herself. Realizing that she was asking for an acceptable way to stop it, the social worker asked the mother if she could accept the doctors approaching her with a recommendation to stop treatment. Mrs. T. said she could not ask them to do that. However, a suggestion that a mutual agreement between physicians and family be made to discontinue the dialysis was acceptable to her.

The next day, the parents, including the father, the physicians, and social worker met and did make a plan to stop dialysis and to do no further procedures of any kind. Oral feedings would be done by the mother as she wished and John would remain in the hospital until he died. The meeting engendered sadness and relief among the family. The renal team continued to visit the mother daily for the remaining three weeks of John's life and provided support to them after John's death.

STRUCTURING ROLES OF THE INTERDISCIPLINARY TEAM

Shared responsibility for patient care usually involves some overlap in team members' roles. For example, the pediatrician, nurse clinician, and social worker listen to the child and parents' reactions, provide information concerning treatment and emotional support. This model of care allows the emotional burdens of treatment to be shared by the team members. In addition, the child and parents have the benefit of contact with a network of professionals who are sensitive to their concerns. At the same time, the roles of the different disciplines must be clearly delineated to avoid confusing families. In our team, the physicians assume the major responsibility for medical decisions and communication of this information to families. The social worker functions in tandem with the physician and provides an ongoing supportive role which can include the role as liaison between the physicians and family. We find that it is often difficult for families to express their concerns directly to the physicians. Parents who feel intimidated by the unfamiliar hospital environment and the physicians' authority are helped to communicate their feelings as in the following case example.

> Angie is the youngest of eight children in a working-class black family who was on hemodialysis. Both parents were involved in her care from the beginning, but the mother was generally more available. Mrs. B., a determined, sometimes angry woman, demanded that her daughter receive the very best medical care in a "white" hospital. Her belligerence was fueled by a fear for her daughter's life, but often made Mrs. B. very difficult for nursing and medical staff to deal with. By contrast, Angie was shy, very quiet, and depended exclusively on her mother to deal with the hospital environment. Gradual but persistent contacts with Mrs. B. established rapport between her and the physicians and social worker. When Angie began dialysis, the mother recognized her own limits and removed herself from the dialysis unit as she became upset and allowed the social worker to provide support to the child.
>
> Despite her initial distress over dialysis, Mrs. B. was able to supprt Angie quite well. During a lengthy but unsuccessful trial with a cadaver transplant, Mrs. B. roomed in the hospital with Angie through several admissions spread over 5 months. Mrs. B. was quite verbal and articulate in her encounters with the social worker but withdrew when the physicians approached her with any news regarding Angie. Unable to overcome this anxiety, Mrs. B. began to use the social worker as "interpreter" between herself and the doctors. She would specifically ask the physicians to outline the problems to the social worker and then wait for the social worker to explain the situation to her. Mrs. B. would often communicate her fears and questions also through the social worker. Mrs. B. gradually developed increasing comfort with the renal team and its ability to understand and act on her concerns about herself and her daughter. Mrs. B. was also open to considering the emotional impact of Angie's treatment. For example, she reported a middle-of-the-night talk between her and her daughter who blamed herself for failing the transplant. Mrs. B. was able to reassure Angie based on the discussion she had with the social worker. Such necessary reassurance was more meaningful to Angie because it was given by her mother. The mother's ability to trust the team allowed her to continue to support Angie who had become increasingly withdrawn and regressed. Mrs. B.'s interventions helped Angie to begin to relate more adaptively to the staff through her extended course of dialysis.

In our team, the nurse clinician also assumes a supportive role with parents and children but has closer contact with the children and the parents concerning their understanding of the disease and treatment regimens. The nurse clinician assumes the important role of helping to clarify children's and families' understanding of procedures and to prepare children for upcoming procedures such as surgery or dialysis. In addition, the nurse clinician helps coordinate the team's patient management with the medical and nursing staff on the hospital divisions. The psychologist's relative isolation from direct patient contact with most families allows him to clarify the team's reactions to patient care and help them plan interventions with families. In addition, the psychologist provides direct service to certain families. For example, some of our children have significant intellectual deficits and learning problems which warrant detailed psychoeducational assessment and communications with the local schools. In addition, the psychologist meets with perspective sibling donors to allow them to discuss their feelings about the donation and to evaluate the nature of their adjustment. Finally, the psychologist assesses the adjustment of more severely disturbed patients and helps plan interventions for these problems. We have found that children's acute emotional reactions can be managed in the pediatric hospital setting with extensive efforts from the team. Some children are also referred to agencies in the communities for psychotherapy.

Although our clinical impressions suggest that a family-oriented approach is helpful to our patients, it is difficult to provide objective evidence of the effectiveness. The majority of our children and adolescents have had reasonable success in coping with life tasks such as school. We have also had good cooperation from our patients in the management of their transplants. In a five-year experience involving 26 transplants, not a kidney has been rejected because of poor compliance with medications. One adolescent experimented with his prednisone and did not take it for a brief period. However, he changed his behavior when the treatment team recognized this and discussed it with him. Some adolescents who had poor compliance before a comprehensive care approach was instituted have improved their compliance in response to the team's efforts.

As our program has expanded and we have added new staff, it has been more difficult to structure team communications. However, our commitment to a family-oriented approach remains very much alive. Our own mutual support and communication continues to be a helpful means of coping with the stressful treatment alternatives for end-stage renal failure.

REFERENCES

1. KORSCH, B. M., FINE, R. N., GRUSHKIN, C. M., and NEGRETE, V. F. Experiences with children and families during extended hemodialysis and kidney transplantation. *Pediatric Clinics of North America*, 1971, 625–637.
2. DROTAR, D., and GANOFSKY, M. A. Mental health intervention with children and adoles-

cents with end-stage renal disease. *International Journal of Psychiatry in Medicine*, 1976, 7, 181–194.
3. DROTAR, D., GANOFSKY, M. A., and MAKKER, S. Psychosocial intervention in childhood renal failure. *Dialysis and Transplantation*, 1979, 8, 73–77.
4. BERNSTEIN, D. M. After transplantation—the child's emotional reactions. *American Journal of Psychiatry*, 1971, 127, 1189–1193.
5. PARSONS, T., and FOX, R. Illness, therapy, and the modern American family. *Journal of Social Issues*, 1951, 31–44.
6. CALLAND, C. Iatrogenic problems in end-stage renal failure. *New England Journal of Medicine*, 1972, 287, 334–336.
7. EISENDRATH, R.M., TOPOR, M., MISFELDT, C., and JESSIMAN, A. G. Service meetings in a renal transplant unit: An unused adjunct to total patient care. *International Journal of Psychiatry in Medicine*, 1970, 1, 53–58.

ADDITIONAL REFERENCES

DROTAR, D. The treatment of a severe anxiety reaction in an adolescent boy following renal transplantation. *Journal of the American Academy of Child Psychiatry*, 1975, 14, 451–461.
KORSCH, B. M., NEGRETE, V. F., GARDNER, J. E., WEINSTOCK, C. L., MERCER, A. S., GRUSHKIN, C. M., and FINE, R. N. Kidney transplantation in children. *Journal of Pediatrics*, 1973, 84, 339–408.
REINHART, J. B. The doctor's dilemma: Whether or not to recommend continuous renal dialysis or renal transplantation for the child with end-stage renal disease. *Journal of Pediatrics*, 1970, 77, 505–506.
VANLEEWEN, J. J., and MATTHEWS, D. E. Comprehensive mental health care on a pediatric dialysis-transplantation program. *Canadian Medical Association Journal*, 1975, 113, 959–962.

10
Observations on Body Image in Renal Patients

SAMUEL BASCH, M.D., FRED BROWN, PH.D., AND WENDY CANTOR, M.D.

The impact that renal disease, its sequelae and complications, and its modern technological treatments have on people so afflicted is protean and pervasive.[1-4] The individual is affected in his internal or psychological being, in his external or social–behavioral being, and in his body or physical being.[5] Although these factors are intertwined, this article will concentrate on the physical being, and more specifically on the body image. For the purposes of this chapter, the body image will be considered as the sum of the mental representations of the body and its organs. The body image does not necessarily coincide with the objective body, e.g., a phantom kidney or the dialysis machine could be experienced as an extension of the body and could be included in it.

In addition to fears of physical deterioration and death, *somatic* preoccupations in renal patients fall into three categories: external disfigurement, alterations in internal body parts and organs, and changes in physiology or somatic functioning.

Concerns about external appearance begin early in renal disease, when there may be incipient, subtle body distortions secondary to fluid accumulations. Later, the dialysis patient is indelibly marked by the surgical reminders of the access site which serves as a stigma or may become invested with special meaning.[6] Indeed, the patient may fix on the access site as the seat of exsanguination or otherwise concern himself with clotting which could deny him his means of survival. Needle marks and other scarred areas become a cause for concern and a focus for feelings of unattractiveness.

SAMUEL H. BASCH, M.D. • Associate Clinical Professor of Psychiatry, The Mount Sinai School of Medicine, City University of New York.   FRED BROWN, PH.D. • Professor Emeritus of Psychiatry (Psychology), The Mount Sinai School of Medicine, City University of New York.   WENDY CANTOR, M.D. • Resident Physician in Psychiatry, New York University Medical Center, New York, New York.

In addition to access site surgery, a variety of medical and surgical procedures which create a sense of internal alteration include uncomfortable peritoneal dialysis experiences or nephrectomy. Nephrectomy may lead to a sense of loss, inadequacy, or incompleteness. Changes in metabolism, overt or subtle, are distressing to the individual. The number of medical and surgical problems fraught by both the disease and the treatment are legion and have a profound impact on the renal patient and his sense of body.

There are a paucity of studies which examine the psychological effects of the nephrological disorders and dialysis on the individual and there has been little attempt to correlate the clinical subjective findings with psychological testing and objective findings.

We studied 16 individuals using a modified version of the House-Tree-Person test. Our modification included person-of-the-opposite-sex and inside-of-a-person drawings[7] as well as selected questions regarding the drawings. For our controls we fell back on the standardized forms done on nonphysically ill people and on comparisons with cardiac, colostomy, cancer, and surgical patients.

We attempted to collect our House–Tree–Person modification from every dialysis patient on our unit using no process of selection. Certain patients were eliminated from the sample because they were physically incapacitated (eyesight, etc.) or otherwise unable to perform the test. We received cooperation from greater than two-thirds of the patients we approached. None of the patients was considered psychotic. All were functioning albeit some in a marginal way not atypical of renal patients.

Limitations of the study included the fact that the total number of patients examined was only 16 and that there was a lack of a specifically determined control group. However, our sample may reflect a typical dialysis unit since we strove to include all patients. Many of the patients excluded were eliminated because of physical disabilities and were not likely to be free from body image problems.

The patients were each given a set of marking pens with a spectrum of ten colors including black. They were instructed to use a pen or pens in any combination or manner they saw fit. They were given five 9" × 12" pieces of blank paper each designated at the top HOUSE, TREE, PERSON, PERSON OF THE OPPOSITE SEX, and INSIDE OF A PERSON. They were instructed to draw pictures depicting the assigned topics marked at the top of the page. Afterwards they were given descriptive questions concerning the drawings.

Our hypothesis before administering the test was that renal disorders and treatment would affect the individual and the quality and content of his drawings. We were interested in observing alterations in cognitive and functional abilities as well as ascertaining if there were alterations in perception, focus, and particularly in body image. The comparison of our results with changes noted in colostomy, cardiac, cancer, and other patients which were specific to their condition and experience would help us to evaluate if there were specific changes in the renal patients. Our results are considered in this context.

All of the drawings were examined and evaluated "blind" by the psychologist who had no previous knowledge of or contact with the patients. In the service of objectivity, psychiatric and other information were withheld until subsequent to the interpretations of the drawings.

The House-Tree-Person consists of both an achromatic and chromatic form, the latter considered by psychologists to tap deeper layers of the personality. The choice of colors has been associated with specific affect,[8] e.g., black and brown occur more commonly in states of inhibition, repression, and possibly regression; blue may indicate some depression of mood tone and a felt need to exercise control; green an attempt to produce feelings of security or relative freedom from threat (except when used for the roof of a house and for foliage); orange as an affective projection of highly ambivalent attitudes in which sensuality and hostility merge; purple as a need for power and possibly reflecting paranoid attitudes, and red as a need for warmth in the environment or as passion. Although we were interested in affect, our findings regarding choice of colors proved to be interesting for reasons later discussed.

The drawings are a reflection of the individual's cognitive functioning and manual abilities. They can also be considered at some level as projections of the person's sense of self and body. The use of the inside-of-a-person test is particularly useful in evaluating individuals with physical disorders.

Other evaluators have viewed these tests in various ways. Buck[9,10] has viewed the house as being endowed with maternal qualities (comfort, safety, security) rather than as a self representation. Certain other evaluators have concluded that particular findings were specific to certain patients, such as colostomy patients[11] or patients with bowel obstruction. The latter were found to have blockages of access to the HOUSE. The PERSON and INSIDE-OF-A-PERSON drawings in open-heart patients exaggerated their focus on the heart[12], etc.

HOUSE

Of all the houses, only one reflected a high level of integration. Half of the houses showed poor perspective or a breakdown in perspective with one side or roof or floor missing or impaired. Several had append-

ages tacked on which one could speculate were equivalents of the dialysis machine, attached to the body as an extension of the body image.
One house appeared as a mass of disorganized blood vessels. Several
patients selected unusual colors (red, pink, orange) which—in context of
the commonly chosen red color in other drawings—one could speculate
as a preoccupation with blood flow related to the blood orientation of the
dialysis unit.

TREE

The trees reflected an exaggerated emphasis on rootedness or firm-
ness in the environment and the need to draw from the ground or outside
source. One could speculate that this could reflect a need for security, a
quest for firm grounding, or a need to extract sustenance from something
external (i.e., dialysis machine, supportive people) or for survival.

Twenty percent of the trees had a split down the middle. Some had
damage and two patients associated that the trees were struck by catas-
trophe or lightning. Others referred to the trees as being sick.

PERSON

Half the drawings were grossly distorted. One third of the patients
showed a split in the body; i.e., a line could be drawn from the top to the
bottom of the figure without touching any parts. Twenty percent of the
patients showed body barrier impairments; i.e., head open, dotted, or
incomplete outlines of the integument.

Several patients had the arms extended to the side in a spread eagle
or cruciform posture. This could indicate a helplessness or possibly reflect
the posture of a reclining dialysand—or both. This also is in keeping with
the exaggerated focus in the drawings on arms and legs—the access sites
essential for survival.

Again six patients selected unusual colors. The two red and three
blue are possibly indicative of the blood environment of the dialysis unit
although the blue may reflect some depression of mood or need for
control. The one yellow drawing was in a patient who had recently
suffered from hepatitic jaundice and who was concerned with his altered
skin color and sclera.

One hundred percent of the PERSON drawings had at least one
finding consistent with a distorted or disorganized concept of body image.

Person of the Opposite Sex

Ordinarily, people draw a figure of their own gender first and then when PERSON-OF-THE-OPPOSITE-SEX drawings are proposed they draw a figure of the other gender.[13] In our sample, seven patients drew their own gender first, five patients drew the opposite gender first, and in four instances the results were questionable or the gender neutral or indiscernible. Of the patients who did not draw their own gender first, all five had sexual problems. The individuals who did draw their own gender first functioned better sexually.

Six men, all with dependency conflicts, drew the person of the opposite sex (a woman) as appearing much larger, stronger and more formidable than the male.

A striking degree of disorganization or disintegration was seen in three drawings.

Half the sample used a red or blue color—again possibly reflecting an artery/vein orientation.

Inside of a Person

Two-thirds of the drawings included kidneys or bladder—not usually drawn in any other condition. Blood vessels and other lines suggestive of blood vessels (if not of tubing—or needles) were seen in five of the patients—also very seldom drawn. Half of the drawings included ribs—again unusual. This finding of ribs is difficult to understand other than considering the ribs serving as a protective cage over the kidneys and other valuable viscera. Perhaps the ribs may reflect the fear of becoming cachectic as the chronically ill patient's disease progresses.

Several patients refused altogether to draw the inside of a person—suggesting their fear of attempting it.

Comments on Drawings

The drawings not selected from a primarily psychiatrically troubled population were more primitive and deteriorated than anticipated. This degree of disorganization and poor perspective is usually seen only in grossly disturbed and psychotic individuals.

The concepts of the body were quite distorted and incomplete. There was no concept of the body as a closed and integrated unit. Parts of the body were missing. There were splits down the middle. Spaces, holes, and impairments were noted. If the abuse of the disease and the extra-corporeal intrusion of the dialysis machine are psychologically damaging, that was certainly evident here.

Patients made obvious attempts to compensate for their feelings of failure physically or feelings of inadequacy. They attempted to compensate or reinforce by drawing double or thickened lines, or by embellishing or adding regeneration to the live figures. Despite this, many drawings revealed an instability or insecurity more marked than was observed clinically in certain patients. The drawings reflected disturbances, and in particular, disturbance of the patients' mental representation of their own bodies far beyond any surface appearance or observable behavior that the staff was aware of.

Some drawings appeared to reflect responses to a feeling of specific traumatic experiences (likely nephrectomy, transplantation, etc.) by associations such as being struck by lightning, etc. The sense of vulnerability was present elsewhere. Many figures were drawn as to appear weak, small, or feeble. Drawings revealed openings and access to the body, almost defenselessly vulnerable. The breaches in the body outline may reflect a lack of a sense of solidity or cohesiveness of the body and its ability to hold together or withstand renal disease or medical incursions. The spread arms defenseless posture was already mentioned. The sense of loss of vitality was present in many renditions of the figure drawings.

Evidence of regression was noted in both the primitive and the infantile quality of some of the drawings as well as in certain specific findings, i.e., the teeth as evidence of oral aggressive regression.

There was evidence of sexual disturbance other than in the person of the opposite sex drawings already noted. Often bodies would be cut off from the waist down or would have no crotch or have an open crotch. Although this bottomless anatomy could reflect the sense of loss of genitourinary, even specifically loss of kidney function, loss of sexual function must also be considered here.

A comment is warranted on the exaggerated use of the color red—selected out of 10 colors. Can this be explained on the basis that these individuals watch their life blood circulate through tubes to a machine and back again? Can it be explained on the basis of this unique situation where the circulatory system becomes externally visible in a situation of potential exsanguination? Or is there another explanation? Perhaps it can be explained on the basis of affect. The inordinate use of the color blue must also be considered here as an indication of pervasive depressiveness not clinically discernible.

These findings are not observed in people not physically ill (standardized controls of House–Tree–Person) nor in colostomy, cardiac, cancer or surgical patients previously studied. These results—

particularly occurring in the combinations observed—appear specific to the uremia—dialysis experience.

Conclusions

The pictures studied suggest deterioration, disorganization, vulnerability, and regression. They also suggest a striking effect on the individual's physical sense, body image, and reactions to the renal situation.

Our patients were not a selected or controlled sample. However, there is no reason to believe they are not typical. Included in our group are people who undoubtedly have organic brain damage, are uremic, or have alterations in their cerebral functioning secondary to metabolic changes from their primary disorders or from complications.

The damage to renal patients may be subtle, insidious, and not readily apparent. The psychological insult may be selective and particularly damaging to body image. It is easy to overlook an otherwise apparently intact individual who may be functioning in all other areas of his life and who may be suffering from a selective if not contained insult to his body ego. There may even be a gross hidden pathologic disturbance not discernible through appearance or behavior.

Future studies should be controlled for illness and current medical status. Studies should be performed preuremia, predialysis, and then at intervals during the course of dialysis taking temporal factors into account. Patients with the same disorders—such as diabetes or collagen disorders—who are physically affected but not on dialysis should be used as controls as well. Only through careful studies can we establish patterns and make generalizations about the specific effects of uremia and dialysis on individuals.

Additionally, baseline drawings could be performed to follow the progress or deterioration of an individual. Drawings could also be used to reveal subtle or underlying disturbances which have not yet surfaced or could be used as prognostic or predictive instruments.

In Summary

These drawings are revealing in that they can visibly document what we already suspect—that renal disease and its treatments have a profound effect on the cerebrum and on the psychological state of the individual. However, these findings underscore the degree of disintegration and disorganization found in some patients and the insidious damage that uremia and dialysis can reek on uremic individuals. The data alert us to look for hidden disturbance, particularly body-image disturbance. They also make us aware that the uremic dialysis experience may have a specific if not unique effect on the individual.

We must keep in mind that these were not primarily psychiatric patients but were individuals functioning in the typical manner of kidney patients. We should remain aware of the handicaps, hardships, and obstacles these individuals have to overcome to carry on in the day to day fashion they do.

REFERENCES

1. ABRAM, H. S. The psychiatrist, the treatment of chronic renal failure, and the prolongation of life. *American Journal of Psychiatry*, 1968, *124*, 10.
2. BASCH, S. H. The intrapsychic integration of a new organ. A clinical study of organ transplantation. *Psychoanalitical Quarterly*, 1973, *42*(3), 364–384.
3. LEVY, N. B. (Ed.), *Living or dying: adaptation to hemodialysis*. Springfield: Charles C Thomas, 1974.
4. LEVY, N. B. The effect of psychosocial factors in the rehabilitation of "The Artificial Man." *Dialysis and Transplantation*, 1979, *8*(3), 213–216.
5. BASCH, S. H. Adaptation to dialysis and body image. *Proceedings of the 5th International Congress on Nephrology*. Krager, Basel, 1974, *Vol. 3*, 211–215.
6. BASCH, S. H. Damaged self-esteem and depression in organ transplantation. *Transplantation Proceedings*, 1973, *5*, 1125–1127.
7. TAIT, C. D., and ASCHER, R. C. Inside-of-the-Body test. *Psychosomatic Medicine*, 1955, *17*, 139.
8. JOLLES, I. *A catalogue for the qualitative interpretation of the H–T–P*. Western Psychological Services, 1952, 7–9.
9. BUCK, J. N. The house–tree–person technique: a qualitative and quantitative scoring manual. *International Journal of Clinical Psychology*, 1948, *4*, 397.
10. BUCK, J. M. The house–tree–person technique: a qualitative and quantitative scoring manual. Part II. *Journal of Clinical Psychology*, 1949, *5*, 37.
11. MEYER, B. C., BROWN, F., and LEVINE, A. Observations of the house–tree–person drawing before and after surgery. *Psychosomatic Medicine*, 1955, *17*, 428.
12. MEYER, B. C., BLACHER, R., and BROWN, F. A clinical study of psychiatric and psychological aspects of mitral surgery. *Psychosomatic Medicine*, 1961, *23*, 3.
13. Levy, S., Projective figure drawing. In: E. F. Hammer (Ed.), *Clinical application of projective drawings*. Springfield: Charles C Thomas, 1967, pp. 91–95.

II
Hemodialysis

11
A Brief Overview of Psychosocial Research on Hemodialysis Patients

FRANZ REICHSMAN

INTRODUCTION

As the title of this chapter states, it will center on the psychosocial aspects of maintenance hemodialysis research. My introduction will be limited to giving my views, or overviews, of the growth of research, of the difficulties encountered in these studies, and of the various objectives or directions these investigations have taken.

It is exactly 15 years since Norman Levy and I began working in Dr. Eli Friedman's service at the Downstate Medical Center to make systematic observations on patients undergoing maintenance hemodialysis. At that time, there was no more than a handful of papers in the literature on the psychosocial aspects in this area, an expression of the fact that only a few psychosomaticists or psychiatrists here and there had been working on dialysis units.

Since then there has been an enormous increase in the collaboration of behavioral scientists and other psychosocial health workers with nephrologists, renal transplant surgeons, and their associates. The result has been a proliferation of studies on the psychosocial aspects of hemodialysis and transplantation.

There has been a remarkable increase in the general *interest* in this field. Published studies number in the many hundreds, as Dr. Patrick McKegney and I noted two-and-a-half years ago when we reviewed much of the world literature in writing a chapter on maintenance hemodialysis for Dr. Eli Friedman's book, *Strategy in Renal Failure*. Dr. Roberta Simmons, who wrote the chapter "Social and Psychological Adjustment of Adult Post-transplant Patients" for the same book, also dealt with a

FRANZ REICHSMAN, M.D. • Professor of Medicine, State University of New York, Downstate Medical Center, Brooklyn, New York. This work was supported in part by NIMH-Psychiatry Education Branch, Grant No. MH 08990-13.

wealth of publications. It would be an oversimplication to state that it was only the dire psychological and social needs of these groups of patients which were responsible for this mushrooming of research, combined with service and teaching as it was. I can think of other new developments in medicine—where patients have similarly urgent needs—which have not brought forth the same degree of interest in and response to psychosocial aspects in those illnesses. A factor of major importance for the development of psychosocial research has been the interest and responsiveness of many nephrologists and transplant surgeons to the psychosocial situation of their patients and their willingness to invite and support the active collaboration of health workers in the psychosocial field. This has been so at our institution and, from what I know, at many other institutions in this country and abroad. A third reason for the great productivity in research is the correct recognition of many workers that hemodialysis and transplantation are excellent opportunities for clinical psychosomatic investigations.

Psychosocial research on patients with end-stage renal failure, being treated with a variety of modalities, has been productive despite the considerable difficulties inherent in it. The difficulties in this field were highlighted for me when a fine North American psychiatrist told me, some years ago, that he had stopped doing research on hemodialysis patients. He added: "There are just too damn many variables in it." However, if many other researchers had not persisted, we would not be writing this book.

Among those who persisted in various countries and have continued, through the years, to make significant contributions are Dr. De-Nour in Israel, Drs. Malmquist and Hagberg in Sweden, Dr. Freyberger in Germany, and, in the United States, Dr. Abram, Dr. McKegney, and Dr. Levy, who—in addition to collaborating and writing original papers—has contributed to the dissemination of information and stimulation of noteworthy discussions (later published) at professional meetings. He has another feather in that cap because of organizing the international conference on which this book is based.

As mentioned, there are indeed a large number of variables to be dealt with when doing psychosocial research in maintenance hemodialysis. At the same time, the groups of patients observed in any *one* study, are relatively small; regrettably, except for a single project which is not completed yet, there have been, to the best of my knowledge, no published studies in which several institutions designed and followed an identical protocol. Furthermore, the patients in the small-group investigations are composed of persons with a variety of illnesses such as chronic glomerulonephritis, polycystic kidney disease, and other renal diseases. In addition, various authors have used different methodologies, making interstudy comparisons a questionable endeavor. Also, many authors have had difficulty in quantifying their observations. Finally, in many patients, the presence of "cerebral insufficiency," a disorder of the intellect, (before *and* during hemodialysis) adds to the complexity of evaluating emotional phenomena.

In this complex situation, it is important that investigators steer between the Scylla, on one side, of giving a "blinding glimpse of the obvious," supported by a wealth of data and statistics, and on the other side, the Charybdis of arriving at broad conceptualizations on the basis of few and insufficiently precise data.

In an overview of the host of publications, it seems important to differentiate the objectives of the wide variety of investigations. Dr. McKegney and I recognized six categories of studies, to which I have since added three more (see Table 1); nevertheless, I do not consider the present list an all-inclusive one. Parenthetically, selection for other treatment modalities such as peritoneal dialysis or "conservative treatment" might also have been included. Although not mentioned in this table, issues in medical ethics are of major importance in this area. The first objective is the description and evaluation of the processes of selection of patients with end-stage renal disease for center hemodialysis.

The second objective has been to identify psychosocial factors that play significant roles in the lives and the adaptation of patients and their families. This includes (1) intrapsychic factors such as the variety of affects and mechanisms of defense and coping; (2) interpersonal relationships of high significance to the patient, and (3) the variety of stresses encountered in maintenance hemodialysis.

As to the second objective, the overall coping and adaptation of patients to maintenance hemodialysis in a sequential pattern, Dr. Levy

TABLE 1
Objectives in MHD Research

1. To describe and evaluate the processes of selection of patients for center hemodialysis, home hemodialysis, and renal transplantation
2. To identify psychosocial factors that play significant roles in the lives and the adaptation of patients and their families
3. To evaluate the patients' cognitive functioning ("cerebral insufficiency")
4. To clarify problems in the interaction between hemodialysis unit staffs and their patients
5. To quantify and evaluate the degrees of rehabilitation of patients on hemodialysis, including attempts to predict patient rehabilitation
6. To describe and assess the overall quality of life of the patients
7. To correlate the patients' psychologic adaptation with social factors (e.g., economic status)
8. To study the body image of the patients
9. To help unit staffs with the day-to-day management of patients

and I described three stages, as did Harry Abram in somewhat different terms. We called the three phrases: "Honeymoon," "Disenchantment and Discouragement," and "Long-term Adaptation." These were observed in a patient population which was at death's door when beginning hemodialysis. Since in many units patients are now placed on maintenance hemodialysis at a somewhat earlier stage of renal failure, the question must be raised whether these stages are still observable. Table 2 shows more specific coping reactions, ranging from successful return to pre-illness functioning, to various degrees of dependence (on Unit Staff and relatives), to denial as a major defense mechanism, to the coping aspects of affects. In any one patient there may be a mixture of these reactions, from time to time. In Table 3 are listed the various stresses on patients undergoing hemodialysis or transplant. Clearly, the importance of any one of these stresses varies from patient to patient and in the same patient from time to time. Not infrequently, two or more of these stresses are present in a given patient at the same time.

A third objective of research in Table 1 is the evaluation of the patient's cognitive, intellectual functioning ("cerebral insufficiency"); it is, of course, of utmost importance to distinguish between intellectual and emotional disturbance and their interplay in these patients.

Table 1 lists three more objectives, the fourth dealing with the clarification of problems in the interaction between hemodialysis unit staffs and

TABLE 2

Coping Reactions of Dialysis Patient

Return to pre-illness function
Dependency
Denial
Coping aspects of affects (communication of
   needs, satisfaction, anxiety, anger, grief,
   depression)

TABLE 3

Stresses of Dialysis and Transplantation

Diet
Dependency
The "Machine"
Physical disability
Social and sexual difficulties
Work and financial difficulties
Fear of living; fear of dying

their patients. This is an area to which Dr. De-Nour has made noteworthy contributions and to which, among others, Dr. Levy and I also paid attention. The next objective has been to quantify and evaluate the degrees of rehabilitation of the patients, including attempts to predict patient rehabilitation. The sixth objective, the description and assessment of the overall quality of life, has too often been dealt with by investigators only in terms of the patient's rehabilitation for employment or housework, without much or any attention to other areas of the patient's life, such as sexual function or gratification, or lack thereof.

See Table 1 for the last three objectives of psychosocial research in maintenance hemodialysis. The first of these has been the correlation between the patient's psychologic adaptation and social factors (for example, with economic status).

Objective number 8, the study of body image of patients undergoing maintenance hemodialysis, has only been dealt with rarely in the literature, until recently. The body image of patients following renal transplantation had received more attention. I am confident that we will be brought up-to-date by the chapters by Drs. Basch and Castelnuovo-Tedesco, on body image in hemodialysis and transplant patients, respectively.

The last listed objective is of particular importance: to help unit staffs with the day-to-day, week-to-week, month-to-month management of the patients. This is a topic of wide scope, ranging from the initial evaluation of the patient, to conferences held by the combined nephrology and liaison staffs (at which either individual patients or general problems may be discussed). It is a topic which includes consultations communicated to an individual nephrologist, nurse, or transplant surgeon, as well as indications for psychotherapy for patients, be it in groups or individually, supportive or uncovering. These broad and vital questions will be dealt with in this book.

In conclusion, I want to point to two research strategies which seem to me to be of particular importance in the near future: (1) psychophysiologic studies, which have been very scarce in the past, and (2) collaborative studies, including transcultural ones. For the second strategy, the first international Conference on Psychological Factors in Hemodialysis and Transplantation gave a splendid opportunity for making a start in this vital direction.

12

Dialysis and Ethics
Be Strong and Trust (Please!)

RICHARD M. ZANER

It is never an easy thing in our times to have the concerns of the philosopher. Not only a sort of "stranger in a strange land," the philosopher is perforce obliged to do what is not usually done within his own native habitat: to gain a real appreciation of the rigors of clinical discipline, but more, to immerse himself in the terribly, and at times for him terrifying, concrete world of human suffering and affliction, thereby to practice his trade of pursuing the raw and disturbing questions of morals, humanity, and understanding. I can only hope that the following thoughts and questions will keep the spirit of that commitment and be actually appreciative of the lives of patients and the labors of clinicians.

There is simply no way for me to treat the moral issues in both dialysis and in transplantation. I shall rather address myself to dialysis; it may be, nonetheless, that these considerations are not unimportant for some of the problems encountered with transplantation.

The medical problems are difficult enough to grapple with—both what leads to end-stage renal failure, and the complications which may be brought on by dialysis itself. But it is rarely the case that even such "medical" problems can be cleanly spliced off from the "psychological" or "social" and "personal" facets of kidney failure and efforts to treat it. Medical contraindications may not be so plain when one seeks to select patients for dialysis, and thus arise the serious questions of finding other criteria by which to select patients. And here, as Abram has pointed out,[1] it is difficult, if not impossible, to separate medical from psychological/ social factors. Recognizing that, furthermore, brings with it some very murky waters indeed: dilemmas proliferate, and the evaluation of selection criteria becomes a formidable task. Concepts such as "cooperativeness," "emotional maturity," or "desire to live" and the like are far from

RICHARD M. ZANER, PH.D. • Easterwood Professor of Philosophy, Southern Methodist University, Dallas, Texas.

clear, and in any case invoke *value* and social worth considerations of the
first order. As it is thus illusory in many cases to try to screen off the
purely medical from the purely psychological, so is it also fanciful to try
this regarding the imperative questions of morality.

But *which* questions are these, and why are they intrinsic to dialysis?
Attention commonly focuses on such as these: allocation of scarce medical resources and the fairness of selection criteria, rising medical costs, the
effect of life-sustaining technology on patients and their families, the
consequences of governmental involvement in the treatment of a particular disease, relations among various health and other professionals, and
similar issues. These alone, however, as Levine urges, make it plain that
dialysis "provides in microcosm an overview of some major ethical issues
in health care today."[2] In few instances is the general pathos of modern
medicine revealed more clearly than in dialysis.

To none of these are there easy or readily available answers. They
remain hotly contested, to the point where it is hardly likely that an
address such as this could hope to settle much, if any, of the obscuring
dust. In any event, I do not propose to enter any of these frays, not
because they are unimportant or uninteresting—quite the contrary.
Rather, I have become fascinated with another cluster of issues presented
by dialysis, one which may well be presupposed by such discussions,
possibly even obscured by them.

Dialysis presents *in extremis* certain phenomena which are deeply
imbedded in most every medical situation of affliction or impairment,
and it is just this dramatic force which is so intriguing. I want to try to
tease it out, as a way of marking out its essentially *moral* fabric—for that is
surely what it is. Doing that will, hopefully, provide a context for understanding more clearly why medicine itself falls, point for point, within the
moral order. If I am not mistaken in these respects, we then have a way of
appreciating just why philosophy, including its concerns for ethics, is a
clear and demanding presence within medicine itself.

Abram underscores a point which even clinical neophytes can readily recognize:

> In chronic dialysis, the matter is not so much one of eternal life but of living
> with the rigors of the medical regimen which may bring about what Unamuno
> termed the "too long" life. And indeed *the* major problem of the dialysand is
> being able to adhere to the dietary restrictions and to tolerate the dependency
> imposed by the treatment, as well as the recurrent physical complications
> associated with dialysis.[1]

This passage is central, for it bristles with ethical issues, though perhaps
not the expected ones.

As is true in most medical situations, but especially is marked in
end-stage renal failure and dialysis, the patient's active participation in

his own treatment and regimen is centrally important for its success. But a common difficulty seems to be how to secure that participation, how to persuade a patient effectively of its critical importance. Somehow, the medical team must "reach" but also "teach" the patient, enjoin him or her to adhere to what must be done. With dialysis patients, however, such efforts are severely complicated by the requisite regimen and what can only be called their recurrent, even methodical encounters with their own deaths.

What Ramsey calls the "mentally punishing procedures" requiring the transplant patient to "die twice,"[3] seems no exaggeration. Indeed, for both the transplant patient and the dialysand, their prolonged lives, as Renée Fox has said, is in truth a "chronic way of dying."[4] Whether this methodical encounter with death be met with intense despair, depression, and even psychosis, or, as in the fortunate few, whether it (as one patient said) "intensifies whatever I am doing . . . sharpens my senses and heightens my appreciation . . . ."[5] there is no way of forgetting for very long that with stark regularity a "kidney machine keeps me alive."[5]

There are two matters to which I want to call attention here, to help elicit the profoundly ethical order presented by dialysis. On the one hand, as Schutz[6] has shown, the veritable mark of everyday life in the common social nexus is what he calls its *taken-for-grantedness*. By way of culturally and socially inculcated typifications, we in the usual course of affairs simply and habitually learn to take hosts of things for granted, as going to be more or less like they have proven to be in the past—at least, for all practical purposes. Only if something does not correspond or conform to our social typifications are we at all alerted to it, called on to take notice of it—and then, our attention is typically directed to settling only what has been unsettled, in order then to proceed with whatever occupies us at the time. Even should we be obliged to change a habit (e.g., using crutches), or alter our life-style (e.g, losing a leg), we typically even then "grow used to it" and our respective stocks of taken-for-granted knowledge remain governed by what Schutz calls the "pragmatic motive" of everyday life.

Illness and impairment, clearly, have a unique way of cutting into that everyday fabric, and things may sometimes radically alter (momentarily or for longer durations). Thus, the man with angina no longer can face even a stairway as once he had; the woman having a cancerous breast removed may now face other people with suspicion at their otherwise innocuous looks; etc. *But how must it be when even the most taken for granted of everything*—that one continues to be alive—not just once but with rigorous regularity, now is no longer able to be taken for granted, so that one's death *looms before one*? Accustomed to being relatively dependent on people in various ways and degrees, and even on things, *how must it be for one to find onself utterly dependent* for one's life on technological devices and sometimes on complete strangers? Whether the machine be regarded as "miraculous monster" or a "hated" machine, dialysands invariably, as Fox says, "view the machine as 'miraculously' rescuing them from death, they also regard it as a constantly fettering, anthropomorphic presence in their life."[7]

This brings me to my second point. The plight of the dialysand is just that he *can no longer take* some crucial things *for granted*, most especially his own continuing to be alive: the very regimen which "rescues"—the machine, the dietary restrictions, the team, the family—at the same time *methodically reminds* the patient of his own unrescueable condition. Furthermore, to the extent that the disease either is, or is experienced to be, something which *befalls* the person, which he could not prevent but must suffer due to the happenings of blind chance or fate, the regularized encounters with his own death and its having to be regularly postponed by means of total compliance with a rigorously enforced regimen and dependence on a machine—this must deeply texture the chronicity of his prolonged living with death by a sense of the *utter injustice* of it all.[8]

This, obviously, is a volatile condition—this continual reminder of the sheer precariousness, indeed the fundamental limits, of one's own life. Given that, it is little wonder that one witnesses the severe "ups and downs" of mood and outlook in such patients, that there is such rapid turnover on the medical team, or that the usual ethical issues have such force for both. For, I want to suggest, that which is the focus of all the efforts, all the costs, all the technology—the dialysis patient— is *himself, in his afflicted condition, one of the root presentations of the moral order,* that is, of what it is to be a moral being, an agent acting in ways which can be called "moral" as well as "immoral." Dialysis uniquely presents that dimension of our lives. For that very reason, furthermore, all of the efforts, costs, regimen, and technologies devoted to the dialysand are in the first instance of the moral order. And in these two presentations—the patient and the medical efforts—one finds the central pathos of medicine mirrored in that of the patient; both present us with an awesome moral dilemma.

Illness, affliction, or impairment are in essence threats or assaults on what constitutes our humanity, as individuals and as members of families and communities. To suffer in those ways is to find one's sense of bodily and personal integrity afflicted, to whatever degree it may be; it is to find diminished one's ability to choose, whether it be one's immediate associates or among alternative courses of action; it is to find oneself willy-nilly dependent upon others, often on strangers, and to one degree or another and whether one particularly likes or has chosen that, or not; it is to find one's sense of oneself impaired, even at times to find onself not knowing what is "good," "appropriate," or "effective" for oneself. Thus, illness and impairment have a unique way of calling attention to the one afflicted. That is, on the one hand, the afflicted person finds himself, however much he may be aware or unaware of this, reliant and dependent on persons, procedures, and technologies he has not self-chosen and on the consequences of which he in all likelihood cannot be expected to be aware. On the other hand, these other persons find themselves (whether by choice or accident, or partly both) counted on, called upon, the focus of the patient's entreaties—again, whether these be trivial or not. *The "fact" of illness or impairment, that is, is a forceful presentation of "value"*; what are taken to be "facts"—whether about "personality," "aggression," or "depression"—are not innocent of serious "values." The collapse of that time-honored distinction is signaled by the central phenomenon of the patient's reliantly calling for help, for a responsiveness by others (often as not, utter strangers). In a word, it is this *call for trust* which is central. But the trust here, and especially with renal disease, is truly fringed with at times bristling regions of ignorance and fallibility, often having nothing to do with either culpable negligence or the "state of the art": about the etiology of renal disease itself, much less the complications (physical and psychological) which seem invariably to ensue with its treatments (transplantation and dialysis), or the difficulties arising from the extramedical contexts of family and community. Where there are even relatively effective "cures," there is then something for the basic "trust" to have a grip upon, and "responsiveness" can be given direction and goal. But, there being no definitive "cure" or apparently much clear prospect for one with renal disease, the "trust" in this case can be, at best, only awkward, and often it seems little more than hopeless. The "appeal" of the patient, intrinsic to his very condition as afflicted, is here a profound pathos evoking a "response" which is equally a moral pathos.

Still, what is unique about medicine is that the appeal issues from one whose very humanity has been afflicted. But, insofar as that is the case, medicine has to do with a person whose very awareness, knowledge, decisions, and the like are diminished, are themselves afflicted. The call and need for trust (not alone from the medical team, but from family and friends) comes from one whose own personal and bodily integrity, whose very life is at stake, and whose own sense of this integrity and life is on the other hand weakened and languishing. Called upon to be morally alert, the patient is nevertheless afflicted precisely in his moral awareness.

With dialysis, I have suggested, those conditions of affliction are brought to a poignant and dramatic focus. To live with the daily assault of awareness of one's own death, to live having to blend the counterattitudes of compliance and collaboration, to be continually aware of the critical impact of one's daily condition upon one's family, to be constantly unable to take it for granted that even one's thirst may be slaked in the hitherto usual ways, to be regularly reminded of the felt injustice of one's condition (having neither chosen it, nor in principle probably having had a hand in choosing it), and to know, sometimes intimately, that other persons may have been denied even this treatment and prolonged life while one receives it—this is surely a potent and awesome moral dilemma! For the medical team, and for the family, furthermore, the situation is similarly unique and potent. For, not only are the members regularly subjected to the entreaties of such afflicted persons, but (at least for now and the immediate future) cannot effectively respond with clear cures, but only by prolonging or helping to prolong their lives, and in that very act reintroducing into the lives of these patients the very thing which gives their entreaties the force and poignancy they have.

Thus, the central phenomenon of "trust"—so essential to patient relations and family ties and so necessary in order to gain the compliant collaboration without which dialysis cannot be more than minimally successful—*presents the medical team with its fundamental problem:* how can the patient be effectively enjoined to adhere to the rigorous regimen native to dialysis? For the family, too, that problem is the continual fabric of daily life. What is it, then, that the patient is being asked to do? To say that the regimen must be followed, I suggest, is to tell the patient that *he must "trust" the medical team.* But, and herewith seems to me the crucial pathos of the dialysand, to express the need for that regimen and thus to ask the patient to trust the medical team is to tell the patient, afflicted already in his or her very humanity, that this affliction must be regularly and methodically borne (with all that implies, including possible psychosis, other medical complications, etc.). Within the very context of this multiple and complex affliction, regularly reintroduced, the dialysand is told that the most important thing which must be done is to follow the regimen with unprecedented rigorousness, i.e., with *courage.* What is called forth, in short, at the heart of these medical transactions, is what classical ethical theorists might well have called "moral strength" or "moral character." This is the case, it needs to be noted, even though many of these patients are notably unable to comprehend just that kind of thing, not to mention what it means to adhere to the rigorous regime of dialysis—even though these persons have been deeply afflicted in their very capacity to comprehend just the kind of moral need and quality their condition requires of them. This is true, too, it might be noted, at an historical time when the sense of what constitutes us as moral beings has been under unprecedented attack, when our moral resources are at severe ebb tide.

The dialysis patient, faced with the unvarying necessity to "trust," "be courageous," and "bear up strongly," as is the family, under a strenuous and difficult regimen—i.e., faced with *the necessity to be moral in the most rigorous sense*—in the teeth of his singularly compelling condition, helps to mark out the essential *conditions of our own humanity as moral beings*, as do few other ailments. His very presence is a clear call for us others to call on our most profound moral resources, for the very nature of end-stage renal failure is that it *presents the medical team, and the family*, not merely the patient, with the fundamental *need to be "of moral strength."* The "support" of a patient, then, is a basically moral phenomenon. Trust, in short, is central, but that can never be taken for granted; it must be cultivated, encouraged, and enabled in all the subtle ways of human intercourse. To "help" such patients is thus always a venture, not always happy, in moral education for all involved. The ethical dimensions of dialysis thus have their root in that ineluctably complex dilemma, and it is, ethically, a profound reminder of our own essential humanity as moral beings. To appraise the quality of such patients' "desire to live," their "cooperativeness," and even their "mental or emotional stability," I must say, is not only to engage in clear value judging, but is also and more disturbingly to have to remind ourselves that in a world dominated by "fact" and approaches to the study of "facts" which seeks to have the rigor of quantitative science, we are nonetheless in the midst of values and the qualitative need to understand them; in this, affliction, and especially dialysis, allows us to catch a glimpse of what ultimately makes us all human, and defines our condition. Only by a clear appreciation of what is fundamentally moral about dialysis, and more generally about affliction, is it possible to address the more usual sorts of ethical issues.

REFERENCES

1. ABRAM, H. S., Psychological dilemmas of medical progress. *Psychiatry in Medicine*, 1972, 3, 51–57.
2. LEVINE, C. Home dialysis and the medicaire GAP, *The Hastings Center Report*, December 1976, 6(6), 5–6.
3. RAMSEY, P. *The patient as person*. New Haven: Yale University Press, 1970, pp. 220.
4. FOX, R. Long-term dialysis programs: new selection criteria, new problems. Adaptation of a case conference at Barnes and Wohl Hospitals, St. Louis, MO.
5. FOSTER, L. Man and machine: life without kidneys, *The Hastings Center Report*, June 1976, 6(3), 5–8.
6. SCHUTZ, A. *The structures of the life-world*. Translated by R. M. Zaner and H. T. Engelhardt, Jr. Evanston: Northwestern University Press, 1973.
7. FOX, R. *The Hastings Center Report*, June 1976, 6 (3), 8–13.
8. SPIEGELBERG, H. Ethics for fellows in the fate of existence, In Peter A. Bertocci (Ed.), *Mid-twentieth century American philosophy: personal statements*. New York: Humanities Press, 1974, pp. 193–210.

13
Prediction of Adjustment to Chronic Hemodialysis

ATARA KAPLAN DE-NOUR

INTRODUCTION

Twelve years ago the number of patients on chronic hemodialysis was limited and treatment was available only to a minority of patients with terminal renal failure. Dialysis units, therefore, had to develop a policy or criteria for acceptance and rejection of patients. Some units attempted to allocate the limited facilities to patients with the best potential for adjustment and survival; in other words, an effort was made to predict adjustment. Although by now there is hardly ever a need to select patients, the importance of prediction of adjustment has not diminished. The ability to predict means that the major sources of stress, as well as the individual's methods of handling these stresses, have been identified. This enables one to plan and carry out meaningful therapeutic interventions. Furthermore, on the basis of prediction, one can decide which of the modalities of treatment will be the least stressful for each patient, i.e., center dialysis, home dialysis, or transplantation. The purpose of the present report is to summarize a series of studies about prediction of adjustment to chronic hemodialysis.

HYPOTHESES

A. There is no global overall adjustment. A patient may adjust or do very well in one aspect and very poorly in another. However, there are relationships between certain aspects of adjustment since these aspects are determined by the same factors and/or because one aspect of adjustment may actually change or influence another.

B. The personality of the patient is the determining factor as far as

ATARA KAPLAN DE-NOUR, M.D. • Associate Professor of Psychiatry, Hadassah Medical Center, Jerusalem, Israel.

adjustment is concerned. Therefore, it is possible to predict adjustment by studying or assessing a patient's personality.

The specific hypotheses about the influence of personality on adjustment were the following:

1. Compliance to the diet is determined by five personality traits (Table 1). No hypothesis was formulated about the relative importance of each of these traits.
2. Vocational rehabilitation is determined by four factors (Table 2).
3. Psychiatric complications (Table 3) are determined by the present level of aggression, the expected increase in aggression that will occur on dialysis (that increase is inversely related to the level of and acceptance of dependency needs), and the defense mechanisms mobilized to handle aggression.

C. Staff attitudes can modify patient's adjustment.

TABLE 1
Personality and Compliance with Diet

Predictive factors
  Frustration tolerance
  Acting out (aggression)
  Denial of sick role
  Gains from sick role
  Obsessive compulsive traits
Modifying factors
  Depression
Other factors
  Locus of control

TABLE 2
Personality and Vocational Rehabilitation

Predialysis level of functioning
Satisfaction with occupation
Dependency needs
Sick role

Locus of control

TABLE 3
Personality and Psychiatric Complications

Level of aggressions
Expected increase in aggression
Methods for handling aggression
  Introjection: depression; suicidal behavior
  Projection: psychotic reactions

METHODS AND PROCEDURES

Patients suffering from terminal renal failure were interviewed a few days to a few months before commencement of dialysis. At the time of the interview, all patients knew about their kidney disease as well as about the planned dialysis. On the basis of this (taped) interview, predictions were formulated separately for each aspect of adjustment. Patients were followed up by a psychiatrist and a nephrologist 6 and 12 months after commencement of dialysis and then at yearly intervals. Details of the predialysis evaluation and follow-ups have been described in previous reports.[1,2]

A total of 100 patients were followed up at least once. The background of the patients was described in a previous report.[2] After the clinical predialysis interview, the patients underwent psychological testing, including the Wechsler-Bellevue Intelligence Test, the Shanan's Sentence Completion Technique (SSCT), and the Rorschach and the Rosensweig Tests. In the present report, only the results of the first two tests are given. Language and literacy problems reduced the sample undergoing predialysis psychological testing. The medical staffs of the units, i.e., the physician in charge and the R.N., were examined by a questionnaire[3] which described their definition of the well-adjusted patient. This questionnaire included 12 items, each composed as a five-point scale, actually describing the staff's expectations about the patient's behavior. In addition, the staff of one unit was studied for acceptance–rejection of patients.[4]

Families were often interviewed, but except for a few they were not systematically studied.[5] It was impossible to assess the influence of the set-up as patients within the same unit did not receive identical treatment. Furthermore, the methods of dialysis changed drastically over the years.

RESULTS

Hypothesis A. Interrelations of Aspects of Adjustment

A positive significant correlation ($\chi_6^2 = 13.81$; $p < 0.05$) was found between compliance to the diet and vocational rehabilitation. In other words, a tendency was found where patients who comply well also achieve high vocational rehabilitation. As will be discussed later, this positive significant correlation is probably due to the fact that some of the personality traits which determine compliance are similar to those that determine vocational rehabilitation.

Positive significant correlations were found between vocational and social rehabilitation (χ^2 = 16.1; p <0.001), as well as between vocational rehabilitation and potency in male patients. It can be suggested that these relationships between various aspects of rehabilitation are, indeed, due to the fact that all aspects of rehabilitation are determined by similar personality traits.

None of the psychiatric complications influenced vocational rehabilitation. A relationship was found between depression and decreased libido and decreased potency. It may be suggested that the decrease in libido and potency is caused by the depression. No relationship was found between depression and impotence.

Some influence of depression and suicidal ideation on compliance was found: Depressed patients complied less well with the diet than predicted. On the other hand, many of the abusers were not depressed.

As could be expected, a significant positive correlation was found between compliance to the diet and survival (χ_2^2 = 10.92; p <0.005). Psychiatric complications also decreased survival significantly. The mortality of the patients who developed psychotic symptoms was significantly higher (χ_2^2 = 9.7; p <0.01) as was that of patients with suicidal ideation (χ_2^2 = 10.89; p <0.005). Figure 1 summarizes the interrelations between various aspects of adjustment.

It seems, therefore, that while there are indeed strong interrelations between some aspects of adjustment, there are no such relations between other aspects of adjustment.

Hypothesis B. Prediction of Adjustment by Assessing Personality

It has indeed been possible to predict various aspects of adjustment by concentrating on the personality traits mentioned.

Table 4 presents the prediction and the actual compliance of the patients and demonstrates that it has been possible to predict compliance. It should be added that in a detailed analysis on a smaller sample, significant correlations were found between two of the traits—level of frustration tolerance and gains from sick role—and compliance. Correlation of each of the other traits separately with compliance failed to reach the level of statistical significance.[6]

Table 5 presents the correlation between prediction and actual vocational rehabilitation and demonstrates that it has been possible to predict vocational rehabilitation. Furthermore, each of the four factors assessed correlated significantly with vocational rehabilitation. Positive significant correlations were found also between predialysis level of functioning and

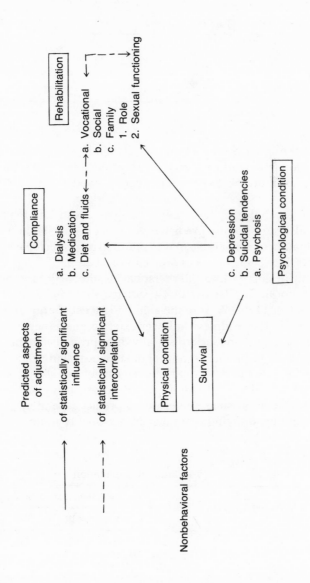

FIGURE 1. Adjustment to chronic dialysis.

TABLE 4
Compliance with the Diet

Predicted compliance	Compliance at last follow-up[a]			
	Good	Fair	Bad	Total
Good	16	8	8	32
Fair	5	29	5	39
Bad	2	1	26	29
Total	23	38	39	100

[a] $\chi_4^2 = 66.80; p < .001$.

each of the other three factors, i.e., dependency needs, sick role, and satisfaction with work. As could be expected, a positive significant correlation was found between dependency needs and satisfaction with work.[7]

The psychological tests, i.e., intelligency tests and the scores of the SSCT, also significantly predicted vocational rehabilitation.[8] Vocational rehabilitation of men (Table 6) was found to be predictable by the following traits: Intelligence, lack of projection and denial (SC, group 2), noninvestment of energy into interpersonal relations (P), and active coping (SC, group 3). The factors that predicted the rehabilitation of women (housewives) (Table 7) were the ability to invest energy in interpersonal relations (P), the readiness to lower external goals (negative correlation with SC, group 1) and lack of socially disapproved activities (−0). It has been possible to predict, at a level of statistical significance, each of the four major psychiatric complications: Anxiety—Table 8; Depression—Table 9; Suicidal risk—Table 10; and Psychotic complication—Table 11.

It has been possible, therefore, to predict separately each aspect of adjustment by studying a number of personality traits.

TABLE 5
Vocational Rehabilitation

Predicted rehabilitation	Rehabilitation at last follow-up[a]				
	I	II	III	IV	Total
I	25	6	3	4	38
II	2	16	2	3	23
III	0	3	5	4	12
IV	0	0	0	22	22
Total	27	25	10	33	95

[a] $\chi_9^2 = 105.42; p < .001$.

TABLE 6
Multiple Regression on Variables Significantly Correlating
with Rehabilitation of Men

	Multiple r	% of explained variance	Explained variance	Pearson's r
IQ	.47[b]	21.8	21.8	.47[b]
SC group 2	.59[b]	35.5	13.7	−.39[b]
P+	.63[a]	39.8	4.3	−.43[b]
SC group 3	.63	40.1	0.3	.38[b]
Education	.63	40.2	0.1	.40[b]

[a] $p < .05$.
[b] $p < .01$.

TABLE 7
Multiple Regression on Variables Significantly Correlating with Rehabilitation of
Women

	Multiple r	% of explained variance	Explained variance	Pearson's r
P+	.47[a]	22	22	.47[b]
SC group 1	.77[a]	59	37	−.45[b]
−0	.81	65	6	−.42[b]
IQ	.87[a]	75.2	10	.29
Education	.87	75.4	0.2	.17

[a] $p < .05$.
[b] $p < .01$.

TABLE 8
Anxiety

	Anxiety at follow-ups[a]			
Predicted anxiety	No anxiety	Moderate anxiety	Severe anxiety	Total
No anxiety	66	6	5	77
Moderate anxiety	7	14	1	22
Severe anxiety	0	0	1	1
Total	73	20	7	100

[a] χ_4^2 46.98; $p < .001$.

TABLE 9
Depression

| Predicted depression | Depression at follow-ups[a] | | | |
	No depression	Moderate depression	Severe depression	Total
No depression	43	10	3	56
Moderate depression	4	23	5	32
Severe depression	0	0	12	12
Total	47	33	20	100

[a] $\chi_4^2 = 91.52$; $p < .001$.

TABLE 10
Suicidal Risk

| Predicted suicidal risk | Suicidal risk at follow-ups[a] | | |
	No	Yes	Total
No	73	10	83
Yes	0	17	17
Total	73	27	100

[a] $\chi_1^2 = 55.37$; $p < .001$.

TABLE 11
Psychotic Complications

| Predicted psychotic complications | Psychotic complications at follow-ups[a] | | |
	No	Yes	Total
No	76	7	83
Yes	6	11	17
Total	82	18	100

[a] $\chi_1^2 = 30.26$; $p < .001$.

Hypothesis C. Staff Attitudes as a Modifying Factor of Adjustment

Although adjustment was found to be predictable, it was found that in all aspects (except for psychotic complications) patients did somewhat less well than predicted. This overestimation of patients' potential for adjustment might be explained by not including some stress factors. On the other hand, the clinical impression has been that in some units the patients do as well as predicted and in other units they do less well. Therefore, the adjustment of the patients in each of the four larger units was studied separately and an analysis was made to find out what percentage of patients did better, as well, or worse than predicted.

Table 12 presents this analysis of compliance. It was found that in some units patients did much poorer than predicted, while in one unit they did even better than predicted. These differences were not so striking in regard to vocational rehabilitation, but in regard to psychological condition, it was found that in one unit the patients did much worse than predicted (Table 13). It was suggested that this (doing less well than predicted) is related to the nurses' attitudes or expectations. In other

TABLE 12
Patients' Compliance

Unit	Percentage of patients complying			Predicted compliance (%)		
	Better than predicted	As predicted	Worse than predicted	Good	Fair	Bad
A	0	65	35	40	40	20
B	9	70	21	13	57	30
C	24	71	5	38	48	14
D	7	67	26	20	53	27

TABLE 13
Psychological Condition

Unit	Percentage of patients in psychological condition			Predicted psychological condition (%)	
	Better than predicted	As predicted	Worse than predicted	Good	Bad
A	0	65	35	75	25
B	4	83	13	61	39
C	5	85	10	71	29
D	4	83	13	60	40

words, when there is intrastaff disagreement about the desired behavior and/or when nurses' expectations are unrealistic, too high, and cannot be fulfilled, patients will adjust less well than predicted.

Table 14 presents the nurses' expectations on the eight adjustment items. The units were found to be different indeed. In Unit A no agreement was found on the important items of compliance and vocational rehabilitation. On the items that describe the expectations in various aspects of the patients' psychological condition, an agreement was found and nurses' expectations were extremely high. In Unit B, no team opinion was found about any item, while in Unit C, team opinion was found about most aspects (including the two compliance items) and expectations were less extreme than in Unit A. It seems, therefore, that the nurses' attitudes, i.e., lack of team opinion or unrealistic expectations, was the cause of the differences in patients fulfilling their potential for adjustment. The ability of the team to form a realistic team opinion seems to be directly linked to the physicians' ability to assess correctly their patients' condition.

TABLE 14
Nurses' Expectations

	Unit A (9 nurses)[a]	Unit B (11 nurses)	Unit C (8 nurses)	Unit D (8 nurses)
Fluid restriction	D[b]	D	2.6	D
R restriction	3.3	D	3.0	3.5
Vocational rehabilitation	D	D	2.6	3.0
Social rehabilitation	4.0	D	D	3.4
Lack of psychopathology	4.0	D	3.0	D
Mood	3.2	D	D	D
Lack of anxiety on dialysis	3.4	D	2.8	D
Nonexaggeration	3.0	D	2.6	D

[a] Range 0–4.
[b] D—disagreement.

TABLE 15
Comparison of Physicians' Assessment to Ours

Unit	Number of points	Percentage of patients doing well in					
		Compliance		Rehabilitation		Psychological condition	
		Phys.	Object.	Phys.	Object.	Phys.	Object.
A	20	40	20	575	15	55	15
B	23	50	15	60	10	90	70
C	21	70	65	40	40	95	70
D	15	45	25	25	25	65	40

Table 16 presents the percentage of patients doing well in the three aspects of adjustment, according to the physician in charge and according to "objective raters." In most units the physicians estimated a much higher percentage as doing well, which indicates denial of external reality. The amount or index of denial was calculated by dividing the two numbers (physicians and objective) (Table 16). The relationship between the realistic team opinion in Unit C (Table 14) and physicians' lack of denial seems clear. Even in the team that had realistic expectations, high emotional involvement in the patients was found. Furthermore, it was found that, to some extent, patients gained acceptance by the staff by being well adjusted patients without severe physical complications, complying fairly well to well with the diet, as well as not having severe psychological complications. However, just to be well adjusted was not sufficient to gain the staff's acceptance. Patients' actual behavior in the unit—good behavior, cooperation, and being interesting to talk to—were important factors in acceptance, while seeking attention and being troublesome led to rejection.

Staff attitudes, therefore, have indeed been found to modify adjustment: Lack of team opinion as well as unrealistic team opinion was found to hamper adjustment. Both attitudes were found to be closely linked to physicians' denial. It was also found that maladjusted patients are more rejected by staff, but at present it is not possible to determine whether maladjustment leads to rejection or whether rejection in any way caused maladjustment.

DISCUSSION

One hundred patients were examined before dialysis and followed up for at least six months. Half of the group was followed up for two years or more. The survival of the patients was on the poor side: By the end of a five-year study, 37 of the patients had died, the majority of them (24 patients) within the first two years of dialysis. The adjustment of the

TABLE 16
Physicians' Denial

Unit	Compliance[a]	Rehabilitation	Psychological condition
A	2.00	5.00	3.66
B	3.33	6.00	1.29
C	1.08	1.00	1.36
D	1.80	1.00	1.62

[a] 1.00—no denial.

group was also on the poor side with only 23 of the 100 patients complying well with the diet and just over half of the group working half-time or more. Thirty patients suffered from moderate to severe anxiety; 53 suffered from moderate to severe depression; 27 were regarded, at some time, as suicidal risks, and 18 had, usually transient, psychotic episodes.

The information gathered over a number of years supported all three basic hypotheses. It was found that patient's personality is the determining factor in adjustment and that adjustment can, therefore, be predicted by concentrating on a number of personality traits. These findings explain some of the difficulties of management with these patients and may also be of value in planning different therapeutic interventions. All of the traits included in the prediction of compliance are, indeed, basic personality traits. In a previous study the difficulties of psychotherapy aimed at achieving change were described.[8] These two sets of observations explain why it is so difficult to improve compliance. By the end of the first six months on dialysis, the majority of patients achieve their level of compliance to or abuse of the diet which they keep to over the years. Neither dynamic psychotherapy nor explanations and threats seem to help in changing this level. Frustration tolerance was found to be highly predictive of compliance and can be increased by hypnosis as well as by behavior modification. The present findings, therefore, suggest that two methods, which so far have not been tried, may improve compliance. The findings indicate that even more can be done to improve vocational rehabilitation: Predialysis regression in functioning should be avoided and satisfaction with work should be increased. This actually means that in order to achieve good vocational rehabilitation of dialysis patients, working with them—including vocational retraining—should begin a long time before commencement of dialysis. Theoretically, this is possible as in most cases patients reach terminal renal failure after a prolonged illness.

Prediction of the psychiatric complications, which was based on the supposed increase in aggression that will occur on dialysis, also seems to indicate that interventions should begin before dialysis. It may be suggested that such psychotherapeutic intervention will not prevent the increase in aggression but may be successful in helping the patients to find ways, other than introjection and projection, for handling aggression, e.g., verbal expression.

The findings about the relationship of patients' personality and adjustment and about the predictability of adjustment indicate also possible approaches to management: Dynamic and/or supportive pshychotherapy once the patients are already on dialysis is likely to be only of limited help. Psychotherapeutic work with the patients should start before commencement of dialysis. The findings also indicate that this work should be "unorthodox" and very flexible. It should be at times dynamic and/or oriented to behavior modification.

The findings also suggest that predialysis assessment of patients' personality might indicate the preferred modality of treatment: Center dialysis, home dialysis, and transplantation are all stress situations, but the sources of stress are somewhat different. It is possible, therefore, to offer the least stressful modality of treatment for each patient. It should be added, however, that so far not enough data has been gathered about the families and which modality of treatment is less or more stressful for each family.

It should be stressed that although all predictions were fulfilled at significant statistical levels, the methods of study should be improved, especially the methods of predialysis evaluation. The data indicates that the elements derived from the sentence completion, together with intelligence tests, may be sufficient to predict vocational rehabilitation but not compliance. It should be added that the scores of the SSCT of patients before dialysis was found to be substantially and significantly lower than those of a matched population.[9] Furthermore, the score changed only little after one year on dialysis. Recently, in another group of patients already on dialysis, the locus of control was found to be higher (more external) than in a normal population. Furthermore, locus of control was found to differentiate between high and low vocational rehabilitation, as well as between compliance and abuse of the diet. It should be checked whether the locus of control, along with the SSCT, actually changes already before dialysis and therefore could be another predictive tool. Without going into more detail of possible methodology, it should be repeated that large predictive studies can be carried out only if so-called "objective methods" replace the clinical interview.

It was clearly found that there is no global or overall adjustment and that patients may adjust well to one aspect and poorly to another. Yet, there are relationships between various aspects of adjustments, e.g., patients who complied well with the diet usually also achieved good vocational rehabilitation. This is understandable as actually similar traits were included in the assessment, e.g., patients with high dependency needs and passive sick role are also those who have many (primary and/or secondary) gains from sick role. It is also understandable that one aspect of adjustment influences another, e.g., that depression lowers compliance. This raises a question about interventions and whether any intervention can be effective if it is not a total push program. It may be suggested that what was found to be true about chronic hemodialysis patients is true also of any other chronically ill patient.

The attitudes of the medical staff were found, indeed, to be a modifying factor. Two types of attitudes were found to be harmful: Lack of team opinion, or in other words, lack of agreement about the expected behavior from "good" patients. This places the patient in a double-bind situation and their adjustment, especially in compliance with the diet, was poorer than predicted. The other antitherapeutic attitude is development of unrealistic expectations which even good patients cannot fulfill. It was found that such an attitude results in patients doing less well than predicted. Furthermore, it was found that these two antitherapeutic attitudes are linked to denial of external reality mobilized by the physicians in charge. The hypothesis that staff attitudes modify patients' adjustment was, therefore, supported. It should be remembered, however, that staff, on the whole, cannot turn a potentially maladjusted patient into an adjusted one. Staff attitudes can allow or disturb a patient from fulfilling his potential for adjustment as determined by his personality. The studies mentioned supported earlier findings both about the differences between units[10] and the emotional reactions of staff.[3,6,11]

Nurses were found to be highly involved with patients, and their acceptance of patients seems to be determined both by how well adjusted a patient is and how well behaved he is. Needless to say, the extreme denial measured in some physicians, as well as the unrealistic expectation of some staffs which are also linked to denial, emphasizes that chronic hemodialysis is stressful also for the staff. Mobilization of denial is an effective defense against the frustrations of dialysis but seems to be harmful to patients.

These findings suggest that something should be done with the staff in order to improve their emotional well-being as well as, indirectly, the patients' adjustment. It is beyond the scope of the present report to go into details of what could, and at some places has been done to improve staff's functioning. Yet, it may be suggested that this indirect approach might be the best for improving patients' adjustment.[11,12]

The data briefly presented were collected over a number of years in chronic hemodialysis units. Such units are very convenient, indeed, for observations and information gathering. Yet, it seems that the findings are actually applicable to other chronic patients: Adjustment should be studied by different aspects and not in global terms; the patient's personality, for example, is an important determinant. Staff reactions can promote adjustment of chronic patients and can also hamper adjustment. It is suggested, therefore, that chronic hemodialysis is but one, though extreme, entity of chronic disability and disease. Hence the extreme importance of improving methods of data gathering.

SUMMARY

Adjustment to chronic hemodialysis, including compliance with the diet, vocational rehabilitation, and psychological condition of patients, was predicted on the basis of patient's personality. The patient's personality was found to be the determining factor as far as adjustment is concerned. Yet, the attitude of the medical staff may be a modifying factor. Two antitherapeutic attitudes were found: lack of team opinion and unrealistic expectations, which are linked directly to the physician's denial. Such attitudes hinder the patients to fulfill their potential for adjustment.

This report summarizes a number of studies and indicates the need to improve methods of information gathering. The findings can serve as an outline for therapeutic interventions with patients and strongly suggest that indirect interventions may be of great value.

It is also suggested that chronic hemodialysis can serve as a model for other chronic diseases, and the findings, therefore, are applicable also to other treatments and disease entities.

References

1. KAPLAN DE-NOUR, A., and CZACZKES, J. W. Personality and adjustment to chronic hemodialysis. In N. B. Levy (Ed.), *Living or dying adaptation to hemodialysis,* Springfield: C. C. Thomas, 1974.
2. KAPLAN DE-NOUR, A., and CZACZKES, J. W. The influence of patient's personality on adjustment to chronic dialysis. *Journal of Nervous and Mental Disease,* 1976, *162,* 323–333.
3. KAPLAN DE-NOUR, A. The influence of physicians' behavior and teams' attitudes on adjustment of chronic patients. In F. Antonelli (Ed.), *Proceedings of the Third Congress of the International College of Psychosomatic Medicine,* Rome, September 1975. Vol. I. Rome: Edizione L. Pozzi, 1977, pp. 120–128.
4. KAPLAN DE-NOUR, A., and CZACZKES, J. W. Nurses' rejection and acceptance of patients. *Mental Health and Society,* 1977, *4,* 85–94.
5. MASS, M., and KAPLAN DE-NOUR, A. Reactions of families to chronic hemodialysis. *Psychotherapy and Psychosomatics,* 1975, *26,* 20–26.
6. KAPLAN DE-NOUR, A., and CZACZKES, J. W. Personality factors in chronic hemodialysis patients causing non-compliance with the medical regime. *Psychosomatic Medicine,* 1972, *34,* 333–344.
7. KAPLAN DE-NOUR, A., and CZACZKES, J. W. Personality factors influencing vocational rehabilitation. *Archives of General Psychiatry,* 1975, *32,* 573–577.
8. KAPLAN DE-NOUR, A., and SHANAN, J. Coping behavior and intelligence in the prediction of vocational rehabilitation of dialysis patients. *International Journal of Psychiatry in Medicine,* 1978, *8,* 145–158.
9. SHANAN, J., KAPLAN DE-NOUR, A., and GART, I. Effects of prolonged stress in terminal renal failure patients. *Journal of Human Stress,* 1976, *2,* 19–28.
10. KAPLAN DE-NOUR, A., CZACZKES, J. W., and LILOS, P. A study of chronic hemodialysis teams: differences in opinions and expectations. *Journal of Chronic Diseases,* 1972, *25,* 441–448.
11. CZACZKES, J. W., and KAPLAN DE-NOUR, A. *Chronic hemodialysis as a way of life.* New York: Brunner and Mazel, 1978.
12. KAPLAN DE-NOUR, A. Role and reactions of psychiatrists in chronic hemodialysis programs. *Psychiatry in Medicine,* 1973, *4,* 63–75.

ADDITIONAL BIBLIOGRAPHY

KAPLAN DE-NOUR, A., and CZACZKES, J. W. Bias in assessment of patients on chronic dialysis. *Journal of Psychosomatic Research*, 1974, *18*, 217–221.
KAPLAN DE-NOUR, A., and CZACZKES, J. W. Emotional problems and reactions of the medical team in a chronic hemodialysis unit. *Lancet*, 1968, *2*, 987–991.
KAPLAN DE-NOUR, A., and CZACZKES, J. W. Professional team opinion and personal bias—a study of chronic hemodialysis unit team. *Journal of Chronic Diseases*, 1971, *24*, 533–541.

14
Hemodialysis, Rehabilitation, and Psychological Support

ALFRED DREES AND EUGENE B. GALLAGHER

INTRODUCTION

Hemodialysis for chronic kidney failure has been technically feasible since the early 1960s, when the devising of shunt access into the patient's blood circulation created the possibility of repetitive dialysis on a long-term basis. With that, dialysis became a life-prolonging technology. In the 15 years since its inception, it has become a widely accepted and practiced technique. Seen in pragmatic cost–benefit terms, it is expensive in resources and money, yet the concomitant benefits are great. Dialysis provides not only sheer life prolongation but also a basis for the patient to live a life which is relatively normal in interpersonal relationships, productive activities, and level of satisfaction. The dialysis patient can, despite the constraints of treatment, achieve a high level of rehabilitation. However, the full potentials of rehabilitation under dialysis have not yet been widely achieved. In this chapter we will examine psychosocial constraints upon the dialysis patient which prevent optimum rehabilitation and discuss psychotherapeutic activities which promise benefit.

This chapter is based upon the collaboration of a psychiatrist (A.D.) and a sociologist (E.B.G.). The psychiatrist has had eight years of supervisory and consultant activity in the dialysis facility at the Medizinische Hochschule in Hannover, West Germany. During this period, he has held regular weekly discussions with members of the dialysis staff and has gained an extensive view of the emotional interpersonal stresses which arise for patients and staff members. The sociologist has studied the expansion of dialysis service at the University of Kentucky. He has also studied the psychosocial adjustment of patients to dialysis, staff

ALFRED DREES, M.D. • Department of Psychosomatics, University of Hannover, Hannover-Kleefeld, German Federal Republic.   EUGENE B. GALLAGHER, PH.D. • Professor of Medical Sociology, Department of Behavioral Science, University of Kentucky College of Medicine, Lexington, Kentucky.

interaction in dialysis units, and political and economic aspects of the mobilization of dialysis resources in several nations.

WHAT ARE THE LIMITATIONS IN DIALYSIS EFFECTIVENESS?

William Ogburn is well known among sociologists for his theory of culture lag.[1] The theory states that human material culture—the tools and physical apparatus of society—changes rapidly because of technological innovation, while the nonmaterial culture—social relationships and ways of realizing goals and values—changes more slowly. Through nonmaterial culture, social behavior becomes adapted to technological change, but the adaptation is slow and imperfect.

As a biomedical innovation with many psychosocial ramifications, dialysis well exemplifies the theory of culture lag. It is a form of high technology which has an indisputable material effectiveness. Dialysis clearly maintains life. Its success lifts it out of the realm of desperate, heroic measures such as heart and liver transplantation. Yet many patients on dialysis lead half lives marked by emotional distress, apathy, and interpersonal strain. The material task of life prolongation is accomplished, but the corresponding nonmaterial task of rehabilitating the patient to a viable life in his social, occupational, and familial contexts has yet to be widely accomplished. While data are available on the sheer extent of dialysis service, little systematic data are available on the rehabilitation of patients. Several studies at particular institutions indicate a high occurrence of emotional problems among patients.[2,3,4] The "soft technology" of psychosocial rehabilitation lags behind the "hard technology" of the dialyzer.[5] With due allowance for the fact that the dialysis process is at present an imperfect, incomplete substitute for the full array of functions performed by the human kidney, we nevertheless believe that more thoroughgoing and better-informed efforts must be made toward the rehabilitation of the patient. To be well directed, these efforts must be based upon an adequate conceptualization of the patient's psychological and social functioning. Patient rehabilitation requires sensitive, sympathetic psychosocial support which complements the biological engineering of the dialysis process itself. The regime of maintenance dialysis is a major life-stress upon the patient, requiring great amounts of time, exposure to treatment risks, and long-term complications; patients on it have been aptly described as "intermittently dying."[6] Stress provokes defensive and adaptive patterns of feeling, thought, and behavior in the patient. An adequate picture of the patient's functioning must thus include an analysis of typical modes of personal response to the dialysis situation.

Patient Psychoreactive States under Dialysis

We present four major psychoreactive states frequently found in relatively clear form among dialysis patients. These states correspond to four developmental stages and may be regarded as ego phases. The major states, and corresponding behaviors, are as follows:

1. Depressive: helpless, pitying, and clinging
2. Aggressive: protesting, compulsively rigid
3. Denying: uncommunicative, pseudostable
4. Adult: mature acceptance of the possibilities, limitations, and risks of life on dialysis

We will briefly describe each state as it expresses itself in relation to dialysis events.

Patients with a long history of disease, and with a correspondingly long period of reduced renal function, may initially experience dialysis euphorically as liberating. But depressive, helpless behavior is also regularly found, sometimes with suicidal tendencies, in the first months of dialysis treatment. Depressive, self-pitying, childlike-clinging behavior accompanied by many psychosomatic complaints is also common among patients after longer periods of dialysis treatment. The frequent violations of drinking and eating restrictions by patients may signify an attitude of oral complaint. Even the rehabilitated patient who manages well for himself through dialysis conducted at home may have depressive crises when somatic complications, marital disruption, or the loss of a job shake his assiduously guarded self-confidence. Great variations in body weight, psychosomatic complaints, or the desire for an early transplant may also indicate a depressive crisis. Somatic complications ending in death often raise the question of suicidal motivation.

Aggressive protesting behavior is seen in some patients in chronic dialysis units, somewhat more frequently in patients in home dialysis training centers, and in home dialysis families who use dialysis as an arena for marital disputes. The general dialysis regime makes precise stipulations in regard both to the patient's diet and the conduct of dialysis treatment. Faced with these exacting expectations, some patients adopt rigid mechanisms of self-control, which have an aggressive tone. Considerable stress is created for family members, nurses, and doctors when this defiant, aggressive attitude prevails.

A group of denying, pseudostable patients is relatively common at chronic dialysis centers. Such patients are typically quiet, factual, and reticent. Staff often mistakenly regard them as phlegmatic and nonreflective, failing to realize how much energy is being tightly bound by the patient's psychic structure under the general stress of dialysis. The patient's bland attitude causes staff to avoid raising vital but anxiety-laden material with him. Such patients may deny the existence of medical complications when they occur. Staff may regard denying patients as unpleasant and poor in establishing contact. They impose neither obtrusive plaintiveness, nor an aggressive and protesting attitude on others. They often are overly demanding in what they expect of themselves, so are in need of particularly careful observation. This attitude is frequently found in home dialysis patients.

The small number of patients with primarily adult mechanisms for controlling their dialysis life is to be found almost exclusively in the group of home dialysis patients. Numerous factors must come together to give a person the strength to cope with the permanent stress of dialysis without decompensating depressively or aggressively, and without denying the seriousness of his situation. Premorbid ego-functioning must be strong. Family and occupational life must be supportive.

The stressful yet routine nature of dialysis treatment evokes characteristic tensions in patient–staff relationships which thwart patient movement toward greater independence and self-activation. Our discussion of "intermediate" psychotherapy below will illustrate how psychodynamically based group discussion among dialysis staff can uncover and resolve such tensions.

LEVELS OF REGRESSION

The basic psychodynamic conflict which pushes the patient into psychoreactive and regressive states is, in our opinion, a conflict between dependence and independence. The patient has, in varying degrees, a mature striving for autonomy and independence. Yet as a seriously ill person, he finds himself dependent upon the expertise and good will of physicians and other health professionals. His dependence upon the dialysis apparatus is particularly dramatic and pronounced. His objective dependency can mobilize preexisting, underlying regressive tendencies. Intertwined with this basic conflict are important variable factors which, taken together, constitute a balance of forces determining the patient's psychoreactive state and level of regression. Our observation of groups of patients in various dialysis facilities has led us to formulate the following four factors which come into play:

1. Premorbid ego strength and family stability
2. Social and occupational security during the period of declining renal function and the beginning of dialysis
3. Extent of patient control over the dialysis process

4. Influence of nurses, doctors, and family members on the patient's access to dialysis

Initially these four causal complexes seemed so interwoven that they did not present themselves as separate categories. It gradually became apparent that the degree to which the patient controls a dialyzer, and the structure and emotional climate of the dialysis program, are particularly decisive in the patient's regaining of self-confidence and autonomy. The dialysis treatment team has a decisive function in this process. We will discuss these relationships in detail.

The artificial kidney, or dialyzer, is a prosthetic device with a vital function for the patient. Without it, he will die. The occasional malfunctions of the dialysis machine reactivate his fears of death and threaten his laboriously erected attitude of wanting to survive. He develops a strong unconscious desire to control his machine, to assimiliate it psychically, so that it can work reliably and exclusively for him without constant, anxiety-fraught attention. It can be said, in general, that a prosthetic device is most effective when it has life-giving and reassuring functions, i.e., when it develops the ego of its user, when it eliminates impediments, and when it works as uncomplicatedly and independently of other persons and care systems as possible.[7] One is reminded of eyeglasses, hearing aids, dentures, and endoprosthetic devices such as cardiac pacemakers. The degree to which a human being can control and take for granted his own prosthetic device determines its value as an instrument for regaining lost powers and for improving the quality of his life.

The patient on a chronic dialysis ward too often feels like an other-controlled, depersonalized entity that is able to survive only as an appendage to the machine and to the sociophysical system in which the machine is housed. He experiences the incomprehensible activities of medical personnel as competently soothing, but also as an infringement of the power to control his own person.

The machine has a life-sustaining meaning for him, but is a prosthetic device in the real sense only to the extent that it liberates him from his dependencies, and returns to him his self-control and self-determination.

At the same time, however, the patient needs the security of expert and competent emergency engineers—nurses, doctors, and technicians. So the problem can be formulated as follows.

Does the patient control his prosthetic device, or is he controlled by the device and its "operating servants"? The peculiar ministruggles that occur on dialysis wards can be comprehended within the context of these salient features which patients present: the familiar-sounding, sometimes openly aggressive tensions, the resigned depressive moods, and poor, uncommunicative pseudorelations with staff.

The fact of the reverse dependence of the dialysis nurse on her patients reinforces the lines of this conflict. The chronically dependent patient becomes "penitently rebellious," and the nurse, who may be insecure in her traditional role in a hierarchical hospital, subjects the patient to increased regressional pressure. The nurse unconsciously tries to force the patient, who developed this attitude as a first step in gaining his independence, back into a depressive, dependent role. A second defense mechanism is also possible: escape by both into mutual isolation, poor communication, and rejection of anxiety-laden dialysis contents.

Figure 1 diagrams the changing relationship of the patient to the dialyzer at varying positions along a "control track." In this conception—not to be understood in a literal quantitative sense—the patient is located on a continuum ranging between polar extremes of dependence and independence. At the pole of dependence, the dialyzer is a dominant, overwhelming force in the patient's life. He experiences it as an external imposed entity, essential to the maintenance of his life but alien to it. It is part of the physical environment and social system of the hospital—all objectively helpful to him, yet complex, remote, and beyond his emotional grasp. At the pole of independence, the patient has psychically assimilated the dialyzer. The machine functions as a true prosthesis. The machine functions as a physiological extension of the patient rather than vice versa. The psychoreactive states set forth above are roughly correlated with locations on the dependence–independence dimension.

THE PATIENT'S STRUGGLE FOR INDEPENDENCE

Patients enter the dialysis regime with various personal histories, which have important implications for their struggle to achieve independence and autonomy. If a patient has been in an extended debilitating phase of declining renal function, his reconstitution at the sheer physiological level—restoration of electrolyte balance, nutritional and fluid stabilization—may require prolonged, intensive staff effort. Once physiologically rescued, he may find it difficult to move toward psychic independence. Rehabilitation is by no means impossible with a patient who has had major renal disease for years, but it requires a new vision by the patient of life's possibilities with dialysis. A positive example is afforded by a 62-year-old diabetic man who moved rapidly into renal failure and dialysis with minimal interruption in his social and family life and in his career as a civil service administrator. His diabetes was of long standing and he had lost his vision to diabetic retinopathy four years previously. He adjusted adequately to that loss and, obtaining readers and other necessary assi tance, continued his demanding job responsibilities. His adjustment to dialysis was similarly quick and thorough. He accepted the necessary burdens. Although he chafed at being hooked to the machine in two lengthy sessions every week, he nevertheless arranged to have important material read to him and to carry on other business during these captive periods.

The start of dialysis treatment typically casts the patient into an unprecedented type of helplessness and dependence. He tries to gain extensive control over his "machine kidney" by depending upon previously learned coping mechanisms, or he remains for a longer period of time in an oral-depressive, clinging stage with a poor prognosis. The next step in his struggle is frequently indicated by defiant protest and complaints. He may try, for example, to have his machine to himself, but at the same time deny his dependence on it, and deny also the precarious balance in which his life hangs.

Machine malfunctions and medical emergencies undermine the patient's sense of security and his perception of himself as a competent survivor. They tend to disturb the process of psychic assimilation of the machine, to prolong regressive states, and to foment conflicts with treatment personnel or family members.

An optimum form of dialysis is that carried out at home, in which the patient keeps his machine in his own dialysis room.[8] Well trained, he dialyzes himself two or three times a week at night. He may even sleep then, because he has experienced reliability of the machine's control system, and because he trusts the medical emergency system that he can call upon in need.

It is possible to correlate the control track of Fig. 1 with levels of

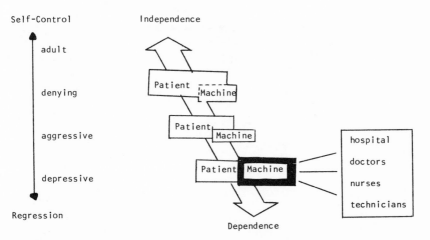

FIGURE 1. Psychic assimilation of the dialyzer.

patient independence under various dialysis treatment systems. This is shown in Figure 2. We distinguish broadly between self-dialysis, which permits greater independence, and medical dialysis, which places the patient under professional control and engenders greater dependency. Full self-care affords the greatest independence, though it is not technically feasible for all patients. Partner care, usually with a spouse or other relative who was trained with the patient in use of the dialyzer, implies somewhat less independence, but the patient is still free of reliance upon professional personnel.

If the patient, with or without help from a partner, is equipped to perform dialysis in his own home, he is more free to schedule his sessions at time suitable to himself—an important factor in attaining maximum independence. In contrast to patients on home dialysis, many patients under medical dialysis cannot maintain employment simply because of job-versus-dialysis scheduling conflicts. Various modes of medical dialysis can also be distinguished from the standpoint of patient independence. When a patient goes to a dialysis center, a single-purpose entity solely for dialysis, he is under professional control. "Center dialysis" is usually a form of "custodial" treatment wherein the patient turns his body over to staff two or three times a week, with little professional concern about his rehabilitation or the broader aspects of his life. Nevertheless, if center dialysis does little or nothing to activate the patient, neither does it demand much of him. Many patients achieve substantial progress under this mode. At a more extreme point in this scale of comparison, the hospital patient receiving dialysis is still more dependent upon, and controlled by, resources outside himself than is the center patient.

Figure 2 correlates patient states, classified between limits of rehabilitation and hospitalization, with positions on the control track. In general the patient's ability to live, love, and work, to participate in social and recreational activities, and to limit the somatic complications of dialysis

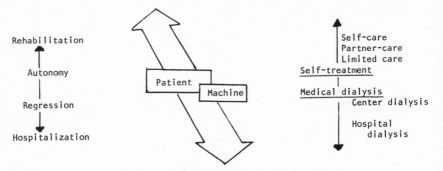

FIGURE 2. Rehabilitation and dialysis control.

are related to the level of autonomy and independence he can achieve in controlling his own treatment. Our observations suggest that psychosomatic manifestations, intrapsychic problems, and family conflicts increase with increasing reliance upon professional resources.

DIALYSIS AND FAMILY STRESS

The marital partner of the dialysis patient has to bear much stress during the predialysis phase of diminishing renal function, and then with dialysis itself. Stress and sacrifice also extend to other members of the family. We have mentioned the stringent limits on food and liquid intake. It is always difficult in family situations to limit the food intake of one member without psychological impact or actual dietary changes for the other members. It is not unusual for patients at home to suck moistened towels, simply to have the sensation of wetness. Such sights also have an impact on the family, perhaps more vivid and tangible than in other serious chronic diseases such as hypertension or diabetes.

The personal sacrifice made by a family member who donates his histocompatible kidney for transplant has been discussed in the popular press and subjected to systematic study.[9] The long-term commitment in time, energy, and care, which a spouse makes in becoming a dialysis partner, is equally great though less dramatic.[10] Sometimes spouses sacrifice more than they emotionally can afford to give and the marital tie is jeopardized. Divorce and marital separation are not uncommon in marriages affected by renal failure and dialysis. Even premorbidly stable marriages can be affected. However, support of a dialysis patient by a stable partner increases his chances of rehabilitation.

The population of dialysis patients is predominantly male, which means that most of the spouses are female. There is a specific set of psychodynamic contingencies related to this which have in repeated instances produced severe marital tensions and conflicts. For the wife to care for her sick husband is a culturally sanctioned role expectation which substantially persists despite many other changes in marital roles. Taken by itself, fulfillment of this expectation would probably produce little conflict. But in a neurotically structured marriage which emphasizes dependent relationships, the wife's role as dialysis partner can create friction. The dominating, hypermotherly wife of a home dialysis patient may after some months find herself with fantasies of murder and a wish for divorce; moreover, careless mishandling of the machine may occur. Dependent husbands who, until they became ill, were able to compensate for feelings of inferiority by high performance in their work or in sports regress to the point where rehospitalization no longer can be avoided. Aside from personality liabilities, there are inherent possibilities for misunderstanding; for example, if a minor disagreement occurs right before a regularly scheduled home dialysis session, the husband may feel that his wife, in establishing blood access, is too rough in sticking the needle in his fistula.

Professional personnel responsible for training home dialysis patients have taken cognizance of these patterns and altered their training procedures. During the initial years of dialysis, it was standard practice to train the wife as the primary partner for home dialysis, and not the patient. This was on the premise that as the patient, the husband was "too sick," and that home care of the sick is a part of the wife's role. Most training centers found that sending the wife home trained for dialysis, with the patient untrained, led to difficulties. This procedure was abandoned as unsound. Now, virtually everywhere, the procedure is reversed; the husband-patient is trained and the wife only receives training, if at all, after the patient is well trained. At some centers, the husband is trained first. Then, as a test of his own comprehension and proficiency, he trains his wife. Training centers also recognize that they have no direct control over the conduct of dialysis—that is, who does what—once the patient is discharged to his own care.

Supportive psychotherapy can be distinctly helpful to the couple when crises occur. It should openly address stress-causing frictions and the functions of both partners in the "dialysis life" of the family. Also effective is special therapeutic attention for the partner, such as treatment of somatic complaints by the dialysis physician, or individual counseling by the psychotherapist. In this case, as in all other marital therapy, one partner must not be played off against the other. Psychoanalytically oriented methods as distinct from supportive methods applied to the partner are not feasible in general, because the exposure of subconscious material places the healthy marriage partner in a special quasitherapist role, or the exposed unconscious conflicts are superadded to marital conflict. Vacation dialysis and temporary relief of the healthy partner from the dialysis situation can be particularly effective for family stabilization when stress mounts.

PSYCHOTHERAPEUTIC POSSIBILITIES IN THE FIELD OF DIALYSIS

A London nephrologist of our acquaintance stated recently that it is the task of the physician to give the renal failure patient a will to live, where he has none of his own. Patients frequently arrive at the hospital in an apathetic, debilitated condition, and they need to be built up motivationally as well as physically. Whatever the value of a positive atmosphere for patients in general, it seems particularly important that the physician and the dialysis team maintain such an atmosphere in their work. This requires, in turn, that they maintain emotional balance in the face of the tedium, the riskiness, and the objective hardship of the dialysis patient's world. Yet dialysis units are commonly the scene of tensions and affective excesses.

> De-Nour and Czaczkes state the reason for this as follows: The special set-up of chronic haemodialysis, with its problems of selection of patients, long-term and intensive contact with a comparatively small number of patients, as well as the new responsibilities that must be assumed by various members of the team, leads to exaggerated reactions.[11]

The working relationships of team members with each other tend to be close-knit, and their level of emotional involvement with the patient is high. For example, patients who violate rules on food and liquid may be unduly censured or rejected; staff expect model behavior from the patients that have been selected, especially since dialysis is a very expensive treatment and other prospective patients may be denied treatment. Staff become possessive and overprotective toward patients. On this basis, patients may be excessively warned about the hazards of transplant or home dialysis, because their treatment track leads the patient away from the staff.

These emotional problems of staff are compounded by traditional rigidities and conflicts in hospital structure. For example, the nephrologist, as physician, expects to function as "captain of the team," yet experienced dialysis nurses frequently have a better grasp of practical aspects of dialysis than does the nephrologist. There may be tense uncertainties about whether the doctor is to function as an all-purpose leader or in a more limited role as consultant and trouble-shooter. Another order of conflict arises between the traditional concept of the "good patient" who is passive and unquestioning, and the independent patient who, in his striving, becomes challenging and assertive.

These manifold sources of tension and conflict on dialysis units taken together form a major impediment to the optimum rehabilitation of the patient and retard his progress along the control track depicted in Figs. 1 and 2. This suggests the value of therapeutic efforts with the staff, rather than the patient directly, in a form of "intermediate therapy" with the goal of promoting a staff climate favorable to patient rehabilitation.

One of the authors (A.D.) has instituted psychotherapeutically directed meetings with dialysis staff. These meetings are not explicit group psychotherapy, and there is no presumption that any participants have personal problems which are to be addressed in the group. Nevertheless, despite the absence of an explicit therapy label, the content of the meetings focuses upon psychodynamic aspects of interactions among staff, and between staff and patients. It is understood and accepted that tensions and conflicts in the dialysis unit involve the interplay of personal and group dynamics within a tightly knit social structure, and that they can be fruitfully explored from this perspective.

Two examples will illustrate the problems considered.

1. A nurse in charge of a patient and his dialyzer is in a bad mood on a particular day. The patient senses this. Feeling highly dependent and vulnerable, he feels that his life is threatened. The nurse, with her bad mood, unconsciously becomes part of his defective body system, instead of the infallible means of rescue. He therefore tries to bind her by many, many requests and questions about the reliability and proper control of the machine. The nurse regards this manifestation of unconscious need on the part of the patient as unreasonable and excessive. She reacts defensively and establishes a vicious circle with cannot be easily interrupted without a new approach to the patient based upon her insight into the situation.

2. Nurses and physicians are regularly caught on both sides of a dilemma in their view of the patient: they signal their hope for more independence in the patient and yet they also express their expectations that he will be a passive, obedient, appreciative "good patient."

Patients are also ambivalently caught on both sides: They indicate their hope of becoming more independent or at least exercising partnership in the control of the machine—and yet they are also possessed by deep dependent, regressive wishes. Staff awareness of the complex interplay of their attitudes with the emotional positions of patients can lead to a more supportive climate.

The goal and strategies of intermediate therapy have been eclectically derived from diverse psychiatric efforts and theories. Intermediate therapy owes much to the work of Rerard and Paumelle in the Thirteenth Arondissement of Paris who, over the past 15 years, have developed a community-oriented, sectorized psychiatry. Therapeutic community concepts, as developed by Maxwell Jones and widely applied in the United Kingdom and United States, are also important.[12] Whatever the external dissimilarities between a psychiatric ward and a dialysis unit, there are common problems grounded in traditionalized, hierarchical role relations, which can be addressed by similar techniques. The applications of Harry Stack Sullivan's interpersonal psychiatry to ward settings by Stanton and Schwartz[13] is likewise a fruitful conceptual approach for dialysis units; distressing episodes which imperil patient progress and staff cohesion can frequently be seen as part of a wider texture of interpersonal tension. Sometimes what appears as an intolerable threat is seen upon closer examination to be a new step of growth for a patient or a new level of professional functioning for a staff member. Balint's psychodynamic conceptualization of doctor–patient communications and relationships is another intellectual root.[14] Finally, the group self-awareness and effectiveness in patient care which intermediate therapy strives for is a form of organizational development which is akin to the methods and goals of the National Training Laboratory in Bethel, Maine,[15] and the Tavistock Institute of Human Relations in London.[16]

PSYCHIATRY AND CHRONIC ILLNESS

Our starting point in this paper was the assertion that the full potential of hemodialysis for rehabilitating renal failure patients has not been achieved. The biomedical technique of dialysis has been developed well beyond the level of psychiatric technique which is available for working with patients undergoing dialysis. More attention to the total psychosocial situation of the dialysis patient—the stresses posed by treatment itself, the impact of machine dependence upon his self-concept, the meaning of dialysis within his interpersonal milieu—is a necessary basis for formulating wise and effective means of support and intervention.

In conclusion, we would like to take a more general viewpoint and argue that psychiatry has much to offer—most of it underdeveloped at present—for the rehabilitation and psychosocial support of a whole range of chronic diseases and conditions. The renal failure patient on hemodialysis, and the kinds of psychiatric activity described, can be regarded as a paradigm for useful involvement in chronic illness more generally. At a confusing time when there are many valid competing models, many professional identity problems, and many new directions in psychiatry, we urge that involvement in chronic illness is a fertile arena for psychiatric attention and development.

The demon of biomedical innovation is producing new technical means of repairing or compensating for damaged senses and muscles, of staving off the malign effects of debilitating diseases, and of replacing the essential vital and vegetative functions of the body. Too often the patient is rescued from death or overwhelming disability only to find that the treatment is very stressful, or that he cannot formulate meaningful personal goals within the scope of his available capabilities. He may have wheelchair mobility but nowhere to go; he may have a fine hearing aid, but nothing in particular that he wants to hear; he may have good occupational potential but be apathetic or resistant toward the prospect of work, as happens frequently with dialysis.

Who has the primary professional responsibility for coping with these discrepancies between the excellence of treatment and the too frequent mediocrity of patient outcome?

The scientists who develop, and the physicians who apply, the biomedical discoveries are, for the most part, interested in treatment excellence far more than patient outcome. Along with other mental health professions, psychiatry can reduce the lag in patient outcome. Although much of this work will occur in university medical centers and other sophisticated medical settings, successful contribution will not depend upon an artificial, exaggerated adherence to a "medical model" of psychiatric functioning. Neither will it rest upon fixed psychopathological concepts of malfunction. Rather, in our opinion, it will draw upon the main body of psychodynamic thinking—those concepts of unconscious defense, psychic energy, and personal growth which have over the past 50 years so greatly illuminated our understanding of what it is to be human. Our foregoing depiction of the dialysis patient will, we hope, serve as a stimulus to a more complete psychiatric concept of the chronically ill or disabled person.

REFERENCES

1. OGBURN, W. F. *Social change*. New York: Viking Press, 1930.
2. BEARD, B. H. The Quality of Life Before and After Renal Transplantation, *Diseases of the Central Nervous System*. 1971, *32*, 24–31.
3. ABRAM, H. S., MOORE, G. L., and WESTERVELT, F. B. Suicidal behavior in chronic hemodialysis patients, *American Journal of Psychiatry*, 1971, *127*, (9), 119–124.
4. WRIGHT, R. G., SAND, P., and LIVINGSTON, G. Psychological stress during hemodialysis for chronic renal failure, *Annals of Internal Medicine*, 1966, *64*, (3), 611–621.
5. GALLAGHER, E. B. Patients, doctors, and policies in renal dialysis, In E. B. Gallagher, (Ed.), *The doctor–patient relationship in the changing health scene*. Washington, D.C.: U. S. Department of Health, Education and Welfare, 1978 (DHEW Publication No. NIH-78-183).
6. BEAVERT, C. S. *Caretakers of the intermittent dying: role strain of a hemodialysis team*. Unpublished Master's Thesis, University of Missouri, Columbia, Missouri, May 1974.
7. HARTMANN, F., and DREES, A. Psychologisch-medizinische aspekte der prothesenmedizin, *Internist*, 1974, *15*, 271–276.
8. BLACKTON, B. Why I am a closet dialysis patient. *NAPHT News*, February 1977, 6–7.
9. SIMMONS, R. G., HICKEY, K., KJELLSTRAND, C. M., and SIMMONS, R. L. Family tension in the search for a kidney donor. *Journal of the American Medical Association*, 1971, *215*, (6), 909–912.
10. FOX, R. C., and SWAZEY, J. P. *The courage to fail* (Second Edition). Chicago: University of Chicago Press, 1978.
11. DE-NOUR, A. K., and CZACZKES, J. W. Emotional problems and reactions of the medical team in a chronic haemodialysis unit. *Lancet*, 1968, 987–991.
12. JONES, M. *The therapeutic community*. New York: Basic Books, 1953.
13. STANTON, A. H., and SCHWARTZ, M. S. *The mental hospital*. New York: Basic Books, 1954.
14. BALINT, M. *The doctor, his patient and the illness*. London: Pitman Medical Publications, Second Edition, 1964.
15. BRADFORD, L., GIBB, J. R., and BENNE, K. *T-group theory and laboratory method*. New York: Wiley, 1964.
16. DICKS, H. V. *Fifty years of the Tavistock clinic*. London: Routledge and Kegan Paul, 1970.

15
Empirical Questionnaire Survey of the Situation of Hemodialysis Patients and Their Partners in Various Dialysis Settings

HUBERT SPEIDEL, UWE KOCH, FRIEDRICH BALCK, AND
JÖRG KNIESS

INTRODUCTION

Systematic studies of the psychological problems surrounding the partners of hemodialysis patients are uncommon, especially surveys with fairly large samples making use of objective methods. We have therefore tried, with the help of a series of standardized tests and a special dialysis questionnaire, to survey both the patients and their partners.

ARRANGEMENT OF THE EXPERIMENT

Questions to be Clarified

1. How do dialysis patients and their partners experience the dialysis situation?
2. What impression do dialysis patients and their partners have of themselves and each other?
3. What changes are made in these impressions in the course of dialysis?

HUBERT SPEIDEL, M.D. • Professor, Department of Psychosomatic Medicine, University of Hamburg, Hamburg, German Federal Republic.   UWE KOCH, M.D., PH.D. • Professor, Faculty of Psychology, Department of Rehabilitation Psychology, University of Freiburg, Freiburg, German Federal Republic.   FRIEDRICH BALCK, M.A. • Psychologist, Department of Psychosomatic Medicine, University of Hamburg, Hamburg, German Federal Republic.   JÖRG KNIESS, M.A. • Psychologist, University of Hamburg, Hamburg, German Federal Republic. This chapter was translated by Richard A. Bird and Kathleen Behnke, Hamburg. The project is sponsored by the German Research Society (Deutsche Forschungsgemeinschaft).

4. What is the connection between measurable personality factors and nature of dialysis experience on the one hand and the conditions of the dialysis situation and the sociodemographic factors on the other hand?
5. What is the nature of the relationships of the couples and its relation to the manner in which the dialysis situation is experienced?
6. What comparison can be made of the various dialysis settings?

Instruments Used

The following questionnaires were used:

1. A 94-item questionnaire on how the dialysis situation is experienced (dialysis questionnaire by Kniess, Budäus, and Speidel) for patients/partners in a hospital unit, and in home dialysis
2. A 12-scale Freiburg Personality Inventory (FPI by Fahrenberg and Selg)[1]
3. The Giessen Test (GT by Beckmann and Richter)[2]—a 6-scale personality inventory in two versions (auto-descriptive and description by another person)
4. A standardized aggression questionnaire (SAF by Koch)[3] with 5 scales
5. A 3-scale questionnaire to register dissatisfaction between couples (Balck)[4]
6. The "quarrel behavior" scale of a questionnaire on work and family situations (KOLA by Koch and Laschinsky)[5]
7. A social statistic questionnaire to record the essential statistical parameters of the dialysis situation

Sample

Patients from four hospital renal units and three private renal units as well as home dialysis patients were surveyed in Bremen and Hamburg. A total of 330 patients were approached. One-hundred-eighty dialysis patients and 150 dialysis partners (57%) returned their questionnaires. There were differences in the returns of the individual questionnaires. The analysis of the patients according to the type of dialysis setting and sex is shown in Table 1. A certain overrepresentation of men (56–44%) is mainly due to the fact that 70% of the patients on home dialysis are men. The average age of the patients is 48.2, of the partners 47.5 years. It is highest in hospital units (51.6) and lowest in home dialysis (42.2). Age is thus a criterion for allocations to the settings. Educational standard cor-

TABLE 1
Analysis of Patients and Partners According to the Various Dialysis Settings and Sex

	Patients				Partners			
Sex	Hospital unit	Private unit	Home dialysis	Total	Hospital unit	Private unit	Home dialysis	Total
Male	19	57	28	104	16	35	10	61
Female	18	52	12	82	14	48	27	89
Total	37	109	40	186	30	83	37	150

responds to the distribution throughout the total population of the Federal Republic of Germany. About 30% of the patients draw pensions premature to age-related retirement. The low proportion of pensioners among the home dialysis patients (12%) is striking by comparison with the private (45%) and hospital unit patients (44%). Occupational degradation as a result of dialysis was an exception. The dwelling situation is worse with private and hospital unit patients, without being associated with differing degrees of satisfaction as regards the dwelling situation between the two groups.

RESULTS

Experience of the Dialysis Situation by the Patient and his Partner ("Dialysis Questionnaire")

The questionnaire was completed by 125 patients and 88 partners. Subjects were asked to respond to questions in seven categories: (1) anxiety in connection with the dialysis; (2) dietary problems; (3) complications and negative physical effects; (4) changes in the interaction between patient and partner; (5) emotional response to weakened social position; (6) the experience of restriction; and (7) withdrawal from social activities.

Anxiety in Connection with Dialysis

Although patients and their partners are convinced that the patient's blood is detoxicated well by the artificial kidney, they worry considerably about the health of the dialysis patient. It is particularly noticeable that these worries—the fear of complications, disquiet because of alarm signals by the machine, and concern for the shunt—are experienced more strongly by the partners than by the patients. The patients have apparently delegated some of their anxiety to their partners or tend more to

TABLE 2
Anxieties in Connection with Dialysis[a]

	Patient	Partner	Patient[b]			Partner			Patient		Partner	
			Z[f]	P[g]	H[h]	Z	P	H	m[i]	f[j]	m	f
Worried about state of health	4.60	5.27[c]					5.27[c]	3.97				
Afraid of complications during dialysis	3.37	3.98[c]	3.83[d]	3.11			4.25[c]	3.57				
Afraid of something serious when unwell	3.19[e]	4.33[d]					4.95[c]	3.57				
Nightmares since being on dialysis	1.81	2.33[d]				4.17[d]	2.75[c]	1.54[c]	1.56	2.15[c]		
Upset by alarm signals from machine	3.12	3.70[d]					4.25[c]	3.57	2.93	3.37[e]		
Worried about shunt	4.30	4.68[e]							3.92[e]	4.82[d]		
Convinced that detoxication of the blood by the kidney machine is good	4.89	4.67[e]					4.42[c]	4.97				

[a] Scales from 1 to 6: 1, does not apply; 6, applies fully.
[b] Significant differences between Z and P are indicated in column Z; significant differences between P and H are indicated in column P; significant differences between Z and H are indicated in column H.
[c] $p < .01$.
[d] $p < .05$.
[e] $p < .1$.
[f] Z, hospital renal unit.
[g] P, Private renal unit.
[h] H, Home dialysis.
[i] m, Male.
[j] f, Female.

deny or displace them than do the partners. Female patients tend rather to give way to anxiety or to suffer more than male patients. While there is hardly any difference in response in dialysis patients between the various dialysis settings, there is among the partners. Differences occur mainly between the partners of private unit dialysis patients and partners of home dialysis patients. Partners of patients on home dialysis obviously feel less anxiety or they manage to displace it better than do the partners of private unit dialysis patients.

Dietary Problems

The patients mostly say that their appetite has improved since they started dialysis. The food that patients and partners eat is similar, although less so for those dialyzed in hospitals. Deliberate diet breaking is admitted by some of the patients, whereas partners deny this. It is least commonly stated that there have been severe complications because of diet breaking by patients in hospital dialysis units and their partners.

Complications and Negative Physical Effects

Sleep impairment of varying degrees, generally since dialysis began and in particular on dialysis days, is reported equally frequently by some patients and partners. Sleep impairment occurs more frequently or to a higher degree in patients on dialysis in private units and in their partners than among those on home dialysis. Whereas the "machine alarm" occurs rarely during dialysis, blood pressure frequently drops. This complication is apparently less frequently registered by partners than by patients. It happens more frequently in private unit dialysis patients than in home dialysis patients and is also reported more frequently by female than male patients.

Partners tend to call upon emergency services more than do the patients. In this respect partners of hospital dialysis patients are clearly different from partners in the other two settings.

Changes in the Interaction between Patient and Partner

The patients have the impression that their partners show greater consideration and that their sense of responsibility has increased since beginning dialysis. They less frequently think that their partners are keeping something from them. Both patients and partners credit each other with being able to put themselves in each other's place. The image of harmony in the partnership is further reinforced by the statement by both patient and partner that the relationship is no less happy during dialysis than it was before.

TABLE 3
Complications and Negative Physical Effects[a]

			Patient[b]			Partner			Patient		Partner	
	Patient	Partner	Z[f]	P[g]	H[h]	Z	P	H	m[i]	f[j]	m	f
Sleep disturbed on dialysis day	3.02	2.92					3.33[d]	2.35			2.38[e]	3.20
Deterioration of sleep since being on dialysis	3.09	3.20		3.45[c]	2.31		3.58[d]	2.68				
Need to call up emergency services at night	1.58	2.00[c]				3.33[d]	2.11	1.63[c]				
Interruption of dialysis by "alarm"	2.64	2.68										
Blood pressure drops during dialysis	3.54	2.8[g,d]		3.95[c]	2.69				3.27	3.91[d]		

[a,b] See Table 2 for explanation.
[c] $p < .01$.
[d] $p < .05$.
[e] $p < .1$.
[f] Z, Hospital renal unit.
[g] P, Private renal unit.
[h] H, Home dialysis.
[i] m, Male.
[j] f, Female.

TABLE 4
Changes in the Interaction between Patient and Partner[a]

	Patient[b]		Patient[b]			Partner			Patient		Partner	
	Patient	Partner	Z[f]	P[g]	H[h]	Z	P	H	m[i]	f[j]	m	f
Impression that partner omits saying a lot of things	2.10	2.56[c]				4.00	2.89[c]	1.95[c]				
Partner doesn't understand properly as he/she can't put him/herself in patient's place	2.05	2.29				3.50	2.52[d]	1.81[d]				
Partner is more considerate	4.82	4.16[d]										
Partner's sense of responsibility increased	4.65	4.13[e]							4.82[e]	4.40[e]	3.78[e]	4.30
Relationship with partner was good before dialysis started	2.75	2.44				5.00[c]	2.33	2.21[c]				
Increased tendency to adopt partner's opinion	2.66	3.33[c]				4.83	3.70[c]	2.60[c]	2.97[e]	2.20[e]		
Thinks he/she must avoid disputes with partner	2.06	2.65[d]										
Now tends more to back down in quarrels with partner	2.25	2.92[c]					3.27[d]	2.50			3.19	2.41[e]

[a,b] See Table 2 for explanation.
[c] p < .01.
[d] p < .05.
[e] p < .1.
[f] Z, Hospital renal unit.

[a] P, Private renal unit.
[h] H, Home dialysis.
[i] m, Male.
[j] f, Female.

By comparison with the patients, the partners feel that they more frequently agree with the opinion of the patients, avoid disputes, and withdraw in quarrels. If we compare the items listed in this table referring to the differences in settings, no differences in the patients are observed. But the discrepancy between partners of patients in different dialysis settings is more obvious. By contrast with hospital and private unit dialysis, in home dialysis the partners' confidence in the patients is obviously greater. The partners of home dialysis patients feel less that the patients are keeping something back from them. They feel better understood by the patients than do the partners of hospital and private unit dialysis patients. Partners of home dialysis patients also feel that they are better able to assert themselves in respect to the patients, that they less easily adopt the patients' opinions, and that they tend to withdraw less in quarrels. Accordingly, they do not idealize their relationship to the sick partner nearly as much as the partners of hospital unit dialysis patients do.

The Weakened Social Position

Many dialysis patients and their partners believe that other people cannot put themselves in their place, that their own ability to assert themselves is severely curtailed, and (this applies in particular to the dialysis patients) that they feel highly dependent on other people. They did not expect sympathy or more consideration from other people.

Home dialysis patients view the future more optimistically than hospital dialysis patients. The lower degree of confidence in the partners of private unit dialysis patients is striking compared to the partners of hospital unit and home dialysis patients. But they suffer less from the idea that other people cannot put themselves in their place. Partners of private unit dialysis patients tend to strongly withdraw when involved in disputes with outsiders. Partners of home and private unit dialysis patients more rarely feel that they are dependent on other people than do partners of hospital unit dialysis patients.

Scrutiny of the sex differences shows that female patients suffer particularly from the fact that, in their opinion, other people cannot easily put themselves in their place.

Experience of Restriction

Most patients and partners report feelings of having to forgo things, of restriction of freedom, and restricted leisure because of the dialysis treatment. Restricted leisure was felt more strongly by patients than by partners. At least some of the patients refer to a decline in their standard of living since they started dialysis and often attribute this to occupational changes. A lower standard of living is reported significantly more often by patients on hospital dialysis than those undergoing dialysis in the other two settings. The feelings that leisure activities are restricted is also more pronounced in hospital dialysis patients than home dialysis patients. Financial restrictions are reported more by male than by female patients. Female partners tend to feel that their freedom is more curtailed than male partners.

Withdrawal from Social Activities

Dialysis patients and their partners reject the assertion that they have been avoiding contact with other people since dialysis started and that their interest in the environment had declined. This applies to partners to a greater degree that it does to patients. Both groups, dialysis patients and their partners, however, report that there has in fact been a withdrawal from social activities since dialysis started. They meet their friends less than they used to; they attend fewer public events and don't frequent as many eating establishments.

Patients on home dialysis more strongly express their interest in the environment than the hospital and private unit patients. They less frequently feel that they were more sociable before dialysis. Even now, after the onset of their illness, they do not attend public events and frequent restaurants and bars less often and accordingly less often have the feeling that they were more sociable before they started undergoing dialysis treatment. The partners of home dialysis patients differ in the same manner from the partners of patients in the other two dialysis settings.

Regarding the differences in sexes, we see that male patients more often avoid restaurants and bars; male partners often report that they were more sociable before their partners went on dialysis than female partners do.

Factor Analytical Findings

Factor analyses were calculated with selected items, separately for patients and partners. The three and four factors identified were:

Patients	*Partners*
Factor 1. Object loss	Factor 1. Object loss
Factor 2. Exhaustion	Factor 2. Stress and depressive reaction
Factor 3. Anxiety/hypochondria	Factor 3. Withdrawl and conflict avoidance
	Factor 4. Deterioration of sexual relations

Male patients exhibit lower figures in the scale "object loss" than do female patients. "Exhaustion" is more frequent in female patients and hospital unit patients than in male patients or patients in the other two dialysis settings. Patients who have been on dialysis a fairly long time display a higher degree of "anxiety/hypochondria."

In the *partners*, there is a trend to show greater "object loss," more in private unit dialysis than in home dialysis and more in women than in men. "Stress and depressive reaction" is more pronounced in hospital and private unit dialysis than in home dialysis. The factor "withdrawal and avoidance of conflict" applies more to private unit partners than home dialysis partners and more to male than female partners.

Personality Questionnaires: Freiburg Personality Inventory (FPI) and Standardized Aggression Questionnaire (SAF)

To throw light on the question of the extent to which the personality profile of dialysis patients and their partners displays unusual phenomena as compared to the normal population, we used the Freiburg Personality Inventory, especially for the aggressiveness area and the standardized aggression questionnaire (SAF of Koch).

Comparison with the control group showed that male patients describe themselves as more nervous, less outspoken, and less self-trusting. Whereas female patients, though also nervous, describe themselves as emotionally more controlled and more self-confident.

Female partners of dialysis patients do not differ from the control group; male partners are more nervous and more easily upset than the control group.

In the five aggression-questionnaire scales, only in the scale "aggressiveness" and/or "competitive behavior" is there a reduction of the scale figures both for patients and partners as compared to the control group.

In comparing dialysis patients with their partners, patients describe themselves as calmer, duller, and emotionally more controlled as well as self-confident and burdening themselves less with feeling of guilt. In the five dimensions of the aggression questionnaire, there is no difference between patients and partners.

Comparison of patients in the various dialysis settings show that, by contrast to home dialysis patients, patients in private units describe themselves as clearly more disturbed psychosomatically, less in need of contact, calmer, and more introverted, as well as more strongly aggression inhibited. The partners of the hospital unit patients characterize themselves—by contrast to the partners of home dialysis patients—as more disturbed psychosomatically, more aggressive, more depressive, more dominant, and more extroverted. The partners of private unit

dialysis patients also describe themselves as more disturbed psychosomatically and more depressive than the partners of home dialysis
patients. In the aggression questionnaire, hospital patients' partners
differ from home dialysis partners by both a higher degree of aggressiveness yet with greater inhibition of aggression.

When interpreting the differences between the settings it must,
however, be taken into account that the allocation of patients to a certain
dialysis setting already depends on certain sociodemographic variables,
so that some of the differences shown here are explained less by the
influence of the setting than by the selection process that has taken place.

The result of further analysis is that patients with a large number of
dialyses exhibit stronger depression, lower extroversion, less self-
confidence, greater reserve, more frequent general psychosomatic disturbances, stronger inwardly directed aggressiveness, greater inhibition
of aggression, and lower aggressiveness than patients with lower number
of dialyses.

Self-Portrayal and Portrayal by Others, as Well as Changes in These in Dialysis Patients and Their Partners (Giessen Test)

A questionnaire which is suitable for use for both self-portrayal and
portrayal by others is Beckmann and Richter's Giessen Test. It contains
the following six scales:

1. Social resonance (attractive, popular, esteemed, able to assert
   oneself, etc.)
2. Dominance (likes to dominate, often involved in disputes, self-
   willed, not readily cooperative)
3. Control (pedantically, orderly, exaggeratedly zealous, constant,
   incapable of being exuberant, talented in dealing with money)
4. Basic mood (depressive vs hypomanic)
5. Permeability (receptive, open to intimacy, openly expressing
   need for love, etc.)
6. Social potency (gregarious, at ease in heterosexual contacts, able
   to form lasting relationship, imaginative)

In our survey, the Giessen Test was used in different versions with
patients and partners: for self-portrayal (both for the present and for the
time before dialysis), and for portrayal of and by the partner, i.e., the
patient portrays the partner and the partner the patient (again both for the
present and for the time period before dialysis).

The changes in the images the patients and their partners had of
themselves and each other, as well as the influence of the dialysis setting
on possible change processes were surveyed.

The fact that the Giessen Test was set in various versions (each person completed the questionnaire from four different points of view) suggested a variance analytical assessment of the data, for each scale a four-factor variance analysis with repeated measurements on two factors was calculated.

- Factor A: Patient vs partner
- Factor B: Dialysis setting (hospital, private unit and home dialysis)
- Factor C: Self-portrayal and portrayal of and by partner
- Factor D: Time (now vs before dialysis)

For factors C and D, repeated measurements are available. The significant results of the variance analyses can be seen in Table 5.

In detail, the following were the results.

1. Scale 1—social resonance. There are significant differences in this respect between self-portrayal of and by the partner. Positive social resonance is used clearly more as a descriptive characteristic in the portrayal of the partner ($p = 0.01$).

In trend ($p = 0.1$), there were also differences for the time of assessment. Patients and partners describe themselves retrospectively as stronger in the sense of a positive social resonance, i.e., they look upon themselves as less attractive than before dialysis.

Over and above this, there is a significant interaction between factor A (patient vs partner) and factor C (self-portrayal and portrayal of and by partner) ($p = 0.01$). Comparison of the four combinations of the two factors shows a tendency towards the positive social resonance's being particularly emphasized by partners in their portrayal of the other partner. It is least emphasized in self-portrayals by partners, i.e., the patients are seen by their partners as especially attractive and esteemed, whereas the partners allocate this characteristic to a lesser extent. An interaction which is also significant resulted from the combination of factors C and D (nature of the report and time to which the description refers) ($p = 0.01$). Closer analysis of this shows that when portraying themselves, patients and partners describe themselves as having positive social resonance before dialysis.

2. Scale 2—dominance. While the major effects do not become significant, the interaction between the first two factors (patient vs partner and dialysis setting) proves to be important. Partners of home dialysis patients and patients on private unit dialysis portray themselves as relatively submissive, whereas home dialysis patients and partners of hospital dialysis patients are by comparison described as dominant ($p = 0.05$).

With the combination of factors A and C (patient vs partner and self-portrayal vs portrayal by partner) it becomes evident that the

TABLE 5
Summary of Variance Analytical Results in the Six Scales of the Giessen Test[a]

	Scale 1 Social resonance	Scale 2 Dominance	Scale 3 Control	Scale 4 Basic mood	Scale 5 Permeability	Scale 6 Social potency
Main effects						
A. Patient vs partner			c			
B. Hospital unit vs private unit vs home dialysis			d			c
C. Portrayal of partner vs self-portrayal	b					
D. Now vs before dialysis	d			b	c	b
Interactions						
A × B	b	c				
A × C		d		d	c	b
A × D						
B × C						
B × D						
C × D	b					
A × B × C						c
A × B × D						b
A × C × D						
B × C × D						
A × B × C × D						

[a] Four-factor Variance Analyses with Repeated Measurement on Factors C and D.
[b] $p < .01$.
[c] $p < .05$.
[d] $p < .1$.

partners' portrayal of the patients and the partners' self-portrayal are described relatively strongly in the aspect of submissiveness, whereas the patient portrayal of the partner is least described in the aspect ($p = 0.06$).

3. Scale 3—control. Comparison of patients and partners shows that, in this scale, partners portray themselves as more controlled than the patients do ($p = 0.05$).

In trend, there are also differences in groups between the three settings, inasmuch as hospital dialysis patients and their partners portray themselves as more controlled than do those in other settings ($p = 0.07$).

4. Scale 4—basic mood. In the scale Basic Mood (hypomanic vs depressive), there are differences merely in factor D (time to which the description refers) ($p = 0.01$), in the sense that the patients and their partners now describe themselves as rather depressive and anxious as compared with the time before dialysis.

5. Scale 5—permeability. As compared to the retrospective assessment, patients and partners now portray themselves as more taciturn, more reserved, and more distrustful ($p = 0.05$).

The interaction between factors A and B (patient vs partner and dialysis setting) also becomes significant. More detailed analysis makes it obvious that hospital and private unit patients display the strongest tendency to portray themselves as distrustful and cautious ($p = 0.05$), whereas home dialysis patients display the least tendency.

6. Scale 6—social potency. In this scale, variance analysis produces a fairly large number of significant findings: Factor B (dialysis setting) displays differentiations of such a nature that the tendency to describe themselves as unsociable is most pronounced in hospital dialysis patients ($p = 0.05$).

The major effect in factor D (time of the description) also becomes significant. Patients and partners are more inclined to describe themselves as socially impotent today than they do in the retrospective assessment ($p = 0.01$).

The interaction between factors A and C (patient vs partner and self and partner portrayal) also becomes significant ($p = 0.01$). Scrutiny of the four possible combinations of the two factors makes it clear that the partners are most strongly characterized by patients under the aspect of social impotence. This emphasis is least in the partners' self-portrayal and in the partners' assessment of the patient.

The subordinate interaction between the first three factors (patient vs partner, dialysis setting, self and partner portrayal) also becomes significant ($p = 0.05$). More precise analysis shows that the strongest tendency to see themselves as socially impotent is in the patient's description of hospital patients' partners and in the self-portrayal of hospital dialysis patients. This tendency is, however, weakest in self-portrayals by home dialysis patients.

Finally, the interaction between factors A, B, and D becomes significant ($p = 0.01$). In this respect, perusal of the combination shows that the descriptions of social impotence are especially pronounced in partners of hospital dialysis patients as related to the present time. Particularly low, by contrast, is this tendency in private unit patients in the retrospective assessment.

Dissatisfaction Problems in the Partner Relationship

This part of the survey was conducted with the dissatisfaction questionnaire designed by Balck and a scale from the questionnaire on the situation at work and in the family (KOLA) by Koch and Laschinsky with results from 109 dissatisfaction questionnaires from the patients' group and 98 from their partners. Only 80 patients' and 67 partners' questionnaires of the KOLA were evaluated.

The four scales used have the following designations:

1. Dissatisfaction with partner's dominance (scale 1, Balck)
2. Dissatisfaction with own dominance (scale 2, Balck)
3. Dissatisfaction with partner's independence and own dependence on him (scale 3, Balck)
4. Couple dissatisfaction (quarrel behavior; KOLA)

Comparison with the Control Groups

As regards the extent of quarrel behavior (KOLA), there is no difference between the dialysis group and the control group. Both patients and partners have, compared to the control group, lower figures in scales 1 and 2. The figures in scale 3 are lower in the partners than in the control group but not in the patients. The whole dialysis group generally describes itself, regarding satisfaction within the partnership, as more satisfied than the control group. This also applies to the separate evaluation of patients and partners.

Comparison of Patients and Partners

The dialysis patients do not differ from their partners on any of the four scales considered.

Dialysis Settings

Both in the patients and their partners, dissatisfaction decreases continuously from hospital through private unit to home dialysis. This applies in the patients to scales 1–3 (Balck); on the other hand, there is in this respect no difference on the couple dissatisfaction scale of the KOLA.

In the partners the corresponding differences tend to be more strongly pronounced: between the hospital and home dialysis settings all mean value differences are significant; between hospital and private unit dialysis there are differences on scale 1, between private unit and home dialysis on scale 2. Quarrel behavior decreases continuously from home dialysis to hospital dialysis. In none of the three settings are there any differences between patients and partners on the four dissatisfaction scales.

Number of Dialyses, Sex, and Age

Patients with a higher number of dialyses tend to more dissatisfaction toward their partners in scales 2 and 3, but not as regards quarrel behavior. Male and female patients do not differ. Differences were found only between male and female partners: male partners are more dissatisfied as regards scale 1–3. The greater dissatisfaction of older patients and partners vis-a-vis younger in the aspects investigated matches the general increase of dissatisfaction in older people[6,7] and presumably does not represent a specific problem of the investigated population.

Variance Analytical Results

Patients

There is an obvious connection between factor 3 (anxiety/hypochondria) of the Dialysis Questionnaire and the dissatisfaction aspects. Patients with relatively strong anxiety and hypochondria in the dialysis situation report low quarrel frequency and quote lower dissatisfaction figures in scales 1–3 than do patients with mean values on factor 3. Patients with relatively little anxiety and hypochondria in the Dialysis Questionnaire also display low quarrelsomeness and low dissatisfaction in scale 2.

Partners

The group with high "object loss" (factor 1) is significantly more dissatisfied than the group with low "object loss" figures. Partners with low figures on factor 3 ("withdrawal and avoidance of conflict") show the highest dissatisfaction figures in all four scales. Partners with high figures on factor 4 ("deterioration of sexual relations") also display, as is to be expected, high dissatisfaction figures in the dissatisfaction scales.

TABLE 6
Variance Analytical Results in the Three Dissatisfaction Dimensions (BALCK) and Quarrel Behavior (KOLA), Comparing Groups with Low, Moderate, and High Degrees of Prominence of Characteristics in Three Dimensions of the Dialysis Questionnaire for Patients

| | Dialysis questionnaire | | | | | | | | |
| | Factor 1 Object loss | | | Factor 2 Exhaustion | | | Factor 3 Anxiety/hypochondria | | |
Dissatisfaction scales	$\bar{X}^a$	GV^b	VA^c	$\bar{X}$	GV	VA	$\bar{X}$	GV	VA
Scale 1: Dissatisfaction with partner's dominance	$\bar{X}$1: 18.89 $\bar{X}$2: 20.57 $\bar{X}$3: 18.68	a: .45 b: .93 c: .42	.69	$\bar{X}$1: 18.26 $\bar{X}$2: 20.90 $\bar{X}$3: 18.33	a: .23 b: .97 c: .25	.38	$\bar{X}$1: 17.30 $\bar{X}$2: 22.17 $\bar{X}$3: 18.61	a: .03 b: .53 c: .13	.07
Scale 2: dissatisfaction with own dominance	$\bar{X}$1: 18.31 $\bar{X}$2: 20.38 $\bar{X}$3: 18.77	a: .33 b: .80 c: .46	.61	$\bar{X}$1: 18.11 $\bar{X}$2: 20.00 $\bar{X}$3: 18.78	a: .33 b: .75 c: .54	.63	$\bar{X}$1: 17.20 $\bar{X}$2: 22.19 $\bar{X}$3: 17.96	a: .01 b: .69 c: .04	.03
Scale 3: dissatisfaction with partner's independence vs own obligation	$\bar{X}$1: 14.41 $\bar{X}$2: 17.10 $\bar{X}$3: 17.32	a: .18 b: .09 c: .92	.20	$\bar{X}$1: 15.22 $\bar{X}$2: 16.97 $\bar{X}$3: 16.19	a: .36 b: .62 c: .68	.66	$\bar{X}$1: 14.33 $\bar{X}$2: 18.00 $\bar{X}$3: 16.39	a: .06 b: .24 c: .45	.15
KOLA "quarrel frequency"	$\bar{X}$1: 13.78 $\bar{X}$2: 15.05 $\bar{X}$3: 12.80	a: .33 b: .24 c: .06	.14	$\bar{X}$1: 14.70 $\bar{X}$2: 12.76 $\bar{X}$3: 13.36	a: .12 b: .37 c: .67	.31	$\bar{X}$1: 13.07 $\bar{X}$2: 15.52 $\bar{X}$3: 12.23	a: .06 b: .50 c: .01	

[a] $\bar{X}$, Subgroup mean values ($\bar{X}$1 = low, $\bar{X}$2 = moderate, $\bar{X}$3 = high scale values).
[b] GV, Comparison of groups (a = 1 vs 2; b = 1 vs 3; c = 2 vs 3).
[c] VA, Probability of the variance analytical F-fraction.

Discussion

If one compares the findings of the dialysis questionnaire for patients and partners, one can presume that the phenomenon of denial in the patients is shown as *delegation* of the patient's anxiety to the partners. This correspondence of intrapsychic and interpersonal processing mechanisms also becomes evident in the FPI. Whereas the patients portray themselves as calmer, duller, more self-possessed, more self-confident, less burdened with feelings of guilt, the partners appear to be more irritable and less tolerant. It can be concluded that irritation attributable to dialysis is delegated, in unconscious interplay, to the partners or it is assumed by them because they, as the ones only indirectly affected by the illness, appear to be fundamentally stronger.

The consequences of this *assignment* for the style of communication between patient and partner can also be gathered from the results of the dialysis questionnaire: the increased consideration shown by the partner towards the patient rather than vice versa and the conflict inhibition of the partner are paid by a general loss of contact and by the general feeling of being under stress. This *distribution* of problems in the relationship between the patient and his partner, problematical though it may appear, provides the patient with an advantage other than that of partial relief from his oppressive problems in connection with dialysis: he is able to see that the partner has developed more sense of responsibility toward him. For the patient, this means *a secondary, partner-related benefit from the illness*. Factor analytical examination shows that the patients and the partners differ in some cases in a characteristic manner with regard to the focus of their dialysis-influenced problems: whereas the patients experience the consequences of their illness (exhaustion) and anxiety about their health preponderate, the problems troubling the partners are of psychic stress, above all, of experience of loss of relationship. While the patients tend to view their partners idealistically with regard to their effect on others, the partners see themselves rather unfavorably in this respect. This also applies to the patient's self-assessment.

Besides these differences, there are, on the other hand, a number of features common to them both: both patients and partners are subjectively burdened by their experiences, which must be qualified as experience of object loss; both differ from the healthy population in respect to their overall aggression behavior, but their competitive behavior, their "aggressiveness," is reduced by contrast to the healthy comparative sample. Apparently, it seems to them that in view of the handicap to be borne jointly, their competitiveness vis-a-vis others is lowered from the start and they are obliged to build up different values and ideals from those of healthy people. That this really is an effect of dialysis is shown by the fact that "aggressiveness" declines with increasing duration of dialysis.

These findings are upheld by the survey of the couples' dissatisfaction: dialysis couples see themselves as more satisfied in comparison to the healthy comparative sample. In the face of the threat from the patient's illness, they are compelled to draw closer together and to establish a lower conflict climate with the partnership, so they succeed, by means of concerted repression,[8] in seeing partner problems as irrelevant. The results of the Giessen Test[9] suggest that this also takes place by means of a decrease of the claim to dominate on the part of the patient, who, because of his problems, sees his partner as especially attractive and esteemed. With increasing duration of dialysis, this form of *joint coping with crises* appears to change inasmuch as it again enables the couple to articulate dissatisfaction, possibly on the strength of a newly acquired *definition of roles.* That the reciprocal satisfaction quoted by the dialysis couples is the result of a common defense process, is vouched for by the results of the GT: both see each other as less attractive, less respected, and less able to assert their points of view than they were before dialysis; they also experience a decline in their social possibilities. The partners obviously feel themselves very restricted in their social realizations by dialysis.

Both the results of the FPI and those of the survey of couple dissatisfaction show that male partners of female patients obviously cope with this situation less well than female partners do. They repress their anxieties at the cost of increased insomnia and a decline in social activities. However, female patients appear, just as do female partners, more restricted in various aspects, such as anxiety, depression, emotional instability, and extroversion. This finding appears, however, as is shown by other surveys, not to state anything about the quality of the female patient's coping with dialysis.[10,11]

The results of the FPI suggest that elderly patients are better able to manage the dialysis situation than younger patients are, if we take the aspects psychosomatic disturbance, self-criticism, and emotional stability as our basis. In the SAF, on the other hand, it becomes apparent that the inwardly directed aggression, i.e., rather self-destructive behavior, is more strongly developed in them. Overall aggression is also more strongly pronounced in them.

Duration of dialysis obviously negatively influences the patients as regards several variables, for example, ability to assert themselves aggressively, the ability to deal with the outside world, and the degree of confidence in themselves, and, in addition, as regards depression and the psychosomatic impairments. These results agree with earlier findings,[10] according to which patients who had been longer on dialysis found it more difficult to adapt to living with dialysis and to come to terms with

166   HUBERT SPEIDEL ET AL

the discrepancy between their activity desires and the limitations dictated by dialysis. Holcomb and MacDonald registered a more favorable life situation two years after dialysis had begun.[12]

In all findings, home dialysis patients appear as the group of patients who were best off overall. For one thing, they most resemble healthy comparative patients in their behavior. As the social data show, this is doubtlessly also a result of the selective allotment of patients to their dialysis settings by the dialysis physicians and by the patients' and their partners' own decision. But the better results throughout for home dialysis patients and their partners also admit the conclusion that this is not solely an effect of selection, but a result of the setting itself. This view is supported by the fact that between hospital and private unit patients, between very similar settings, in other words, there are differences of varied natures in the results which can scarcely be explained by selection processes in every case. After all, the assumption that selection processes alone could be considered responsible for the differences above all between home dialysis and the other two settings, would contradict the finding that elderly patients cope better with the dialysis situation, even if at the cost of increased (and inwardly directed) aggression, in view of the fact that the home dialysis patients in our sample are on the average fairly young. The increase in difficulties with duration of dialysis also contradicts the hypothesis that selection processes alone can be held responsible for the better psychosocial situation of the home dialysis patients, because the average duration of dialysis in our sample is longer for home dialysis patients. The factors of age and number of dialyses, would thus lead us to expect comparatively worse results from home dialysis patients, whereas the opposite is in fact true.

Taken together, the results not only confirm that dialysis is, in various respects, a heavy burden for the patients. It appears particularly noteworthy that the partners are also affected in many respects just as much, if not more, by dialysis. A conclusion that can be derived from this study is that offers of psychotherapy to hemodialysis patients, which are quite generally useful and necessary, should bear reference to the partners.[13] In particular need of therapy are the patients on hospital dialysis and private unit dialysis and their partners, to whom priority should be given.

REFERENCES

1. FAHRENBERG, J., and SELG, H. *Freiburger Persönlichkeitsinventar (FPI)*. Handanweisung. Göttingen: Hogrefe, 1970.
2. BECKMANN, D., and RICHTER, H. E. *Giessen Test (GT)*. Handbuch. 2nd Ed. Bern, Stuttgart, Wien: Huber, 1975.
3. KOCH, U. *Der standardisierte Aggressionsfragebogen (SAF)*. Arbeitsbericht des Teilprojektes C 1, SFB 115, 1974, 11–20.

4. BALCK, F. Fragebogen zur Erfassung der Unzufriedenenheit zwischen Freundes- und Ehepaaren. Unpublished manuscript, Hamburg 1975.
5. KOCH, U., and LASCHINSKY, D. Ein Fragebogen zur Erfassung der Situation and Arbeitsplatz und in der Familie (KOLA). *Psychologie und Praxis*, 1979, *4*, 165–173.
6. BLOOD, R. O., and WOLFE, D. M. *Husbands and wives: the dynamics of married living.* Glencoe, Illinois: The Free Press, 1960.
7. MILLER, B. C. A multivariate developmental model of marital satisfaction. *Journal of Marriage and the Family*, 1976, 643–657.
8. MAURIN, J., and SCHENCKEL, J. A study of the family unit's response to hemodialysis. *Journal of Psychosomatic Research*, 1976, *20*, 163–168.
9. SPEIDEL, H., KOCH, U., BALCK, F., and KNIESS, J. Problems in interaction between patients undergoing long-term hemodialysis and their partners. *Psychotherapy and Psychosomatics*, 1979, *31*, 235.
10. SPEIDEL, H., BAUDITZ, W., BUNGER, P., FREYBERGER, H., v. Kerekjarto, M., and Ramb, W. Beitrag zur Psychopathologie der Dauerdialysepatienten. *Verh. Dtsch. Ges. Inn. Med.*, 1970, Vol. *76*, 1040–1042.
11. LEVY, N. B., and WYNBRANDT., G. D. The quality of life on maintenance hemodialysis. *Lancet*, June 14th, 1975.
12. HOLCOMB, J. L., and MACDONALD, R. W. Social functioning of artificial kidney patients. *Social Science and Medicine*, 1973, *7*, 109–119.
13. SORENSEN, E. T. Group therapy in a community hospital dialysis unit. *Journal of the American Medical Association*, 1972, *221*(8), 899–901.

ADDITIONAL BIBLIOGRAPHY

KOCH, U., BALCK, F., and SPEIDEL, H. Psychische Probleme bei Haemodialyse-Patienten und ihren Partnern. *Bericht über den 31. Kongress der Dtsch. Ges. Psychol.*, Mannheim 1978. Göttingen: Hogrefe, II. Halbband S. 450.
SPEIDEL, H., v. KEREKJARTO, M., KNAUF, B., and PROBST, P. Psychische und psychosoziale Probleme bei Prothesenträgern: ein Vergleich zwischen Patienten mit Hüftendoprothesen, künstlichen Herzklappen und unter chronischer Hämodialyse. *Med. Psychologie*, 1975, *2*, 127–158.
SPEIDEL, H. Die Arbeit des Psychomatikers in Dialysezentren. *Der Krankenhausarzt*, 1976, *49*, 10, 648–651.
SPEIDEL, H. Zur psychischen Situation des Pflegepersonals bei Heimdialyse und Heimdialysetraining. *Therapiewoche*, 1976, *26*, 7, 1043–1047.
SPEIDEL, H., BALCK, F., and KOCH, U. Psychische und psychosoziale Probleme der chronischen Hämodialyse. *Therapiewoche*, 1978, *28*, 43, 8262–8279.
SPEIDEL, H., KOCH, U., and BALCK, F. Dauerdialysebehandlung und Patient. In F. W. Albert, G. A. Jutzler, H. Kreiter, and G. Traut (Eds.), *II. Symposion der Nephrologischen Arbeitsgruppe Homburg-Kaiserslautern*. Wiss. Information der Freseniusstiftung, 1978, Beih. *5*, 13.

16

Denial and Objectivity
in Hemodialysis Patients
Adjustment by Opposite Mechanisms

BRUCE H. BEARD AND TOM F. SAMPSON

Patients with end-stage renal disease are treated with hemodialysis to extend their lives and maintain their physical status so they may function as effective and productive family and community members. Patients generally attempt to adjust to their illness and treatment as though they were in an improving state and often as though they were hardly ill at all. One of the mechanisms of defense they use is denial which makes it appear as though they see themselves as being only marginally ill and marginally handicapped while also appearing to negate the fact they have a serious and usually irreversible disease. The use of denial has been widely documented[1-5] and has been accepted as an almost universal defense in dialysis patients. This study revealed evidence which indicated that patients in addition to denial make equal use of the adaptive process of objectivity facing reality in an undistorted manner. By believing and yet denying they have a serious illness, dialysis patients use two diametrically opposite adjustment mechanisms. Furthermore, this study revealed one other significant phenomenon, specifically, that patients shift back and forth from denial to objectivity in a rapid and never-ending fashion. It is believed that this balanced shifting between these two divergent strategies is essential for harnessing the adaptive strengths of both defenses for use in surviving the prolonged ordeal of life on dialysis.

BRUCE H. BEARD, M.D. • Clinical Professor of Psychiatry, University of Texas Southwestern Medical School, Dallas, Texas. TOM F. SAMPSON, M.S. • Clinical Psychologist, Southwestern Dialysis Center, Dallas, Texas.

METHOD AND RESULTS

Psychological Test Data

The following psychological test data concern the use of denial by dialysis patients and indicate that denial is often overdetermined and overdriven. Our study consisted of 26 patients, 15 females and 11 males, ranging in age from 21 to 74 years. They were administered the Bell Adjustment Inventory, Multiple Affect Adjective Check List, and Purpose in Life Test to assess adjustment in a broad range of life situations, quantify affective states, specifically depression, anxiety, and hostility, and measure attitudes toward purpose in living. The Bell Adjustment Inventory yields scores on five separate adjustment measures, (1) home, (2) health, (3) social, (4) emotional, and (5) occupational, reflecting the individual's subjective impression of his adaptation in these specific areas. Results of the Adjustment Inventory indicated the patients saw themselves as adjusting significantly better than the norm group in home, social, and occupational areas. In emotional adjustment the difference was not significant, although weighted in the direction of better emotional adaptation in the dialysis group. Only in health adjustment did the dialysis patients rate themselves significantly more impaired than the norm group, indicating greater problems and dissatisfaction with health. The overall results indicated that despite obvious and persistent difficult life circumstances in which the patients found themselves, dialysis patients reported adjustment levels, with the exception of health, better than those in the norm group who suffered no major physical disability or life-threatening illness.

The Multiple Affect Adjective Check List (MAACL) provides measures of three clinically important affects: anxiety, depression, and hostility. Results of the Affect Check List showed statistically significant differences between the study and norm groups in the direction of the dialysis patients reporting less anxiety and hostility.[6] On the depression scale the difference between the two groups was not significant, but was weighted in the direction of the dialysis patients reporting fewer feelings of depression.

The Purpose in Life Test is an attitude scale constructed from the orientation of Victor E. Frankl's logotherapy and indicates positive and negative feelings regarding purpose in life. The test also assesses certain attitudes about death. The Purpose in Life Test revealed the dialysis group perceived purpose and meaning of life greater than that of the norm group. The implication was that dialysis patients had a heightened appreciation of life, perhaps from being exposed to the possibility of an untimely death. For them the value in being alive at the moment was intensified. Living seemed more worthwhile and they felt they had more to live for in spite of their impaired state.

In summary, the findings of the Adjustment Inventory and Affect Check List indicated the use of denial to an overdetermined degree. The dramatic results of the Purpose of Life Test reflected the unusual life experiences of the dialysis patients. In some respects, their heightened purpose in living also suggested the use of overdenial of untimely death.[3]

An example of a patient who utilized overdetermined denial was a woman whose initial reaction to renal failure was principally objective and was manifested by extreme, explosive anger and frustration. She felt her whole life had fallen apart. She avoided dialysis for many months and insisted on working instead. She thought, "I'll work as long as I can and then die." Later, after starting dialysis, denial replaced objectivity and she came to believe herself capable of living a full productive life, one who would outlive most others with illnesses such as heart disease or diabetes. She saw herself as a healthy, active individual who swam, hiked, and did whatever she wished. She planned for years ahead, took a course in cake decorating, and planned to open her own business catering weddings and parties. She even saw herself operating a chain of catering businesses and buying real estate in addition. Her plans included adopting children and rearing them without a husband. She felt she was not ill, not impaired, and thanked God for the healthy organs she had that functioned well. Fortunately, she had retained sufficient objectivity to acknowledge that staying well did mean staying on dialysis.

Clinical Data

Having learned from personal observations and psychometric test data that dialysis patients when left to their own dictates tend to present themselves in an overdetermined denial fashion, it was decided to devise an interview that would enable the patients to ease off of their denial stance and reveal other attitudes concerning their lives and their illness. A structured format was developed that began with open-ended broad questions concerning the patients' first reactions to learning they had renal disease and ended with inquiries into their thoughts of death and the likelihood of an untimely death. There were 15 basic questions. In some instances the sequence of the questions was altered as the interview progresses, but in all interviews the information sought by each question was elicited. The questions were as follows:

1. When were you first aware of having kidney disease?
2. At that time, what did you think about having kidney disease?

3. What changes did having kidney disease make in your life?
4. When did complete renal failure occur?
5. What did you think when you learned that renal failure had occurred?
6. What changes did complete renal failure make in your life?
7. What did you think when you first learned you were to go on dialysis?
8. What changes has dialysis made in your life?
9. Has renal failure and dialysis altered your future life's plans?
10. Do you consider yourself ill at this time?
11. Has renal failure made any changes in your family?
12. How far into the future do you plan?
13. Has renal failure and dialysis altered your religious beliefs and your relationship to God?
14. Has renal failure and dialysis changed your thoughts about death?
15. Do you feel optimistic or pessimistic about improvement?

Parenthetically, it should be stated that following the patient interview, the most significant relative was interviewed. This data was used to determine concurrence by the relative with the information given by the patient. It was found that there was close correlation between the relatives' opinions about the patients' attitudes and the data the patients gave about themselves.

The answers to each question were rated by both investigators independently as to whether they demonstrated denial or objectivity. The answers were then grouped into eight subgroups: those relating to (1) predialysis, (2) dialysis, (3) illness, (4) family change, (5) future planning, (6) religious beliefs, (7) death, and (8) improvement. The questions relative to predialysis were predominantly answered with denial. Those relative to dialysis and its effects were also weighted on the side of denial. Attitudes as to whether the patient considered himself ill or not were weighted on the side of denial but the spread was not great. Attitudes about changes in family life were weighted on the side of denial. At this point a shift occurred in the interview responses. The questions that focused on the change in the patients' relationship to God showed a significant number of objective answers. There was also a significant number of objective answers to questions related to death. The most revealing question was the one concerning future planning. The patients in a ratio of three to one objectively stated that life was so uncertain, not only as to length but also as to quality, that they did not plan beyond a short range and in some instances not beyond one day ahead. The final question relative to optimism versus pessimism about improvement revealed an almost even distribution between denial and objectivity. Thus, the structured interview showed a statistically significant incidence of conscious objectivity on the part of the patients when the interview progresses in a step-by-step manner to personal attitudes about future planning, relationship to God, and death.

An example of a patient who used sharply focused objectivity almost exclusively was a woman whose reaction to first learning she had kidney disease was, "Why is it happening to me? It would have been better if I had died." She was depressed then and is still depressed at times now. Following renal failure her life completely reversed itself from one in which she was an active, gregarious, verbal person to one in which she was severely restricted physically and had problems in communicating because of a hearing loss. Starting on dialysis seemed unreal and her first dialysis was recalled as a terrifying experience. Gradually she adapted but life became centered around her dialysis schedule. Trips, whether long or short, had to be planned around it. Tickets to entertainment events were not bought in advance because she could not know if she would be well enough to attend. Her future plans of being a college librarian or teacher were discarded. "Now I plan only a day at a time." As to the length of her life, the patient was not sure she would live to see her grandchildren born. Instead, she projected herself into the future on a short-term basis. Fear that she might not be alive for long kept her from planning long range. Only occasionally did she and her husband casually mention the possibility of some future plan, but the patient feared that even if alive she might not be able physically to participate in any planned activity. Death was seen as an imminent event, something that could happen to her at any time. Each day she woke and thought, "I see I'm still here." This patient's viewpoint of her existence was so predominantly objective that life appeared harsh and filled with negative apprehensions from which there was little relief.

Even more enlightening than overdetermined denial and harsh objectivity, this study by use of the structured interview revealed a phenomenon of rapid shifting from objectivity to denial and vice versa. The patients seemed totally unaware of this shifting process. The ease with which they made the shifts was felt to be indicative of the fact that this mechanism was well intrenched and the patients engaged in shifting not only in verbal speech but also in private thinking. An example of rapid shifting was observed in one patient who stated he accepted without difficulty learning he had renal failure and adapted his life easily to dialysis. In the same sentence he stated that the knowledge of his impaired health bothered him so much that he constantly had to put it out of his awareness. He acknowledged dialysis stood between him and death and this knowledge held in check his recurring desire to discontinue dialysis and return to unfettered days doing as he pleased. He acknowledged a wish for no restraints in his life only to counter with the statement that he came for dialysis automatically without a reluctant thought. Concerning planning, the patient in a single sentence stated he could see himself functioning well forever, then abruptly stated he could not picture himself ten years ahead, or even five, and actually he lived from day to day, not planning at all. When pressed further about future planning, he stated he did not plan to marry anytime soon, then stated he could not see himself ever marrying or raising children. In addition, he denied being ill but could not explain how that belief was compatible with his not seeing himself existing in the future. Concerning death, he stated he would live as long as anyone and backed up this belief by stating that he would live a normal life for years. In the next sentence, he stated that in the past he saw himself living a normal life but now he never planned ahead because he did not know how he would feel the following day.

DISCUSSION

The use of overdetermined denial by dialysis patients is of importance because it is a means by which patients protect themselves from what they consider devastating and intolerable knowledge. But denial alone would likely lead patients to disastrous noncompliance and even treatment refusal.[7] Objectivity, however, serves the purpose of constant orientation of the patients in relation to life and death and keeps them on dialysis and cooperative with the rigors of the treatment program. But objectivity alone would undoubtedly lead to overwhelming discouragement and disabling depression.[1,8] Rapid shifting from objectivity to denial and vice versa creates a balance between the two opposite defenses. This shifting phenomenon was judged to be the mechanism that gave flexibility and strength to what would otherwise be an unadaptable choice of one defensive stance or the other.

A word about needs of the patients which the staff is in a position to help meet. It is easy to augment the denial portion of the patients' awareness of themselves. Our study indicated that staff could be of additional service if they would also support the patients' objectivity and reality facing by making appropriate inquiries that would encourage them to verbalize, however briefly they may choose, the fact that they give frequent consideration to their needs for a relationship to God, their reluctance to plan into the future, and their thoughts about the uncertainty of the length of their lives. Since objectivity is an integral part of the patients' adjustment mechanism, supporting their often unstated objective reality facing efforts will facilitate their adjustment strength and can be a vital part of staff function. The technique utilized in the structured interview of narrowing discussions with patients in a step-by-step fashion from broad issues to highly focused references to planning, religious involvement, and thoughts of life and death can be the means of providing this support of the patients' objectivity.

CONCLUSION

This study concluded that denial and objectivity are of equal importance as adaptive mechanisms. Denial is more apparent and is utilized more often in the patients' interpersonal contacts, but in their own private thought worlds, the patients are objectively aware of the reality of their illness and its effect on their lives. In addition, the patients shift at a rapid rate from objectivity to denial to fill alternately the need for reality orientation and the need for reduction of anxiety generated by reality facing. It was concluded that the balanced use of denial and objectivity and the ability to shift rapidly from one to the other enables the patients to make the best possible use of both mechanisms and prevents their becoming locked into an inadaptable use of one defense without the other. This intricate phenomenon was considered to be an essential aspect of the adaptive ability that dialysis patients demonstrate and gives their ego structure the flexibility required to survive. All told, there is no question but that the adaptive strength that most dialysis patients show is extraordinary and those of us who work in this area of medicine stand in awe at the ability of these patients as they struggle, oftentimes successfully, to maintain lives of acceptable quality.

REFERENCES

1. ABRAMS, H. S. Psychiatric reflections on adaptation to repetitive dialysis. *Kidney International*, 1974, 6, 67.
2. GLASSMAN, B. M., and SIEGEL, A. Personality correlates of survival in a long-term hemodialysis program. *Archives of General Psychiatry*, 1970, 22, 566.
3. BEARD, B. H. Fear of death and fear of life. *Archives of General Psychiatry*, 1969, 21, 373.
4. SHORT, M. J., and WILSON, W. P. Roles of denial in chronic hemodialysis. *Archives of General Psychiatry*, 1969, 20, 433.
5. DE-NOUR, A. KAPLAN, SHALTIEL, J., and CZACZKES, J. W. Emotional reactions of patients on chronic hemodialysis. *Psychosomatic Medicine*, 1968, 30, 521.
6. FISHMAN, D. B., and SCHNEIDER, C. J. Predicting emotional adjustment in home dialysis patients and their relatives. *Journal of Chronic Diseases*, 1972, 25, 99.
7. McKEGNEY, F. P., and LANGE, P. The decision to no longer live on chronic hemodialysis. *American Journal of Psychiatry*, 1971, 128, 267.
8. LEFEBVRE, P., NORBERT, A., and CROMBEZ, J. C. Psychological and psychopathological reactions in relation to chronic hemodialysis. *Canadian Psychiatric Association Journal*, 1972, 17, 9.

17
Use of Fantasy for Conflict Resolution in the Pediatric Hemodialysis Patient

TOM F. SAMPSON

INTRODUCTION

Assessment of the emotional status and characteristics of children is frought with considerable difficulty primarily because of the fact that we have only limited access to their private worlds. This seems certainly to be the case with children in end-stage renal disease. Our major avenue for assessing such psychological material is through verbal interchange, as we would have with adults. Level of cognitive development in children often times all but precludes obtaining such information through verbal interview. Additionally, research data[1] indicates fear, a condition frequently noted in children on hemodialysis, generates massive inhibition which attenuates the experience of fear and may obliterate it. As a result, often times information regarding the psychological status of children is obtained from those close to them, i.e., parents, teachers, etc., as well as observation of the children's behavior. Even these methods, however, do not allow us access to the private world of the child which would provide a more direct knowledge of their perception and relation with the world.

The problem just described was encountered in a previous study[2] wherein it was determined that children in renal failure and on hemodialysis had two distinctive, behaviorally overt, methods of interacting and coping with their environment. Briefly, one group was noted to display withdrawn behavior, particularly in the dialysis setting, while the other group of children showed a coping mechanism characterized by a readiness to interact with others. Through interviews with the parents and observations of the children's overt behavior, it was determined that these children experienced conflicts in their lives and consequently had periods of anxiety that were observed to interfere with their daily living.

TOM F. SAMPSON, M.S. • Clinical Psychologist, Southwestern Dialysis Center, Dallas, Texas.

Lacking, however, was a clear knowledge of the nature and origin of these children's conflicts as well as their resolution or attempted resolution because of the fact there was only limited access to the child's inner thoughts. What we had were, for the most part, observations of children's behavior made by us and others close to them.

The most direct method of determining the nature of these children's conflict was considered to be by tapping their private thoughts or their fantasy. It is contended by investigators[3,4] that the themes about which an individual characteristically fantasizes are loosely but directly correlated with his typical pattern of overt behavior. The relationship exists because both overt behavior and fantasy themes are each in their way determined by current concerns—concerns created by goal striving efforts that potentiate corresponding themes and fantasy. A casual observation of the child in renal failure and on dialysis would show the strength and intensity with which the child's condition is frequently in the foreground of his awareness. Thus was the rational for relying on fantasy to provide direct information about the child's inner world and particularly the conflicts he experiences surrounding his illness and dialysis.

The study had three major emphases. The first was to determine if elicited fantasy from children on hemodialysis would provide direct and relevant information regarding the child's perception of his world as well as how he related to it. The second issue was an effort to determine whether, and if so how, the fantasy life of the child interfaced with his day to day relations with the environment. The third investigated issue was the examination of the fantasy productions of the two groups of children, i.e., withdrawn versus engaging, to determine if, as the case with their behavior, they utilized fantasy differently.

Each of the children in the previous study as well as children admitted to the hemodialysis unit since that time were interviewed in depth being asked to produce outcomes to fairy tale stories presented to them (there were numerous variations of the method), and also to respond to unstructured and semistructured psychologic instruments.

Briefly, the results showed a construction of fantasy themes related to the immediate influences and activities of these children's lives. The scope of the themes were dominated in form, by productions concerning fear and aggression. Additionally, the elicited fantasy productions revealed the world being seen as confusing, hostile, and threatening. The one other theme that dominated in frequency was dependency. Knowledge of these psychological states was believed to be provided through the medium of elicited fantasy, and further would not have been easily accessible through direct observation or standard interview with the child. The results further indicated that the fantasy productions of these children served a control function by regulating the expression of the child's conflict by binding the psychic energy associated with the conflict. Consequently, the fantasy productions in the children were seen as utilization by them of resolving their conflicts by creative use of problem solving. With regard to the third emphasis of the study, it was revealed that there were differences in the ways in which the children utilized their fantasy production—primarily in the area of total number of fantasy productions and greater emphasis on dependency themes by the withdrawn group.

METHOD

The population of the study consisted of 23 children ranging in age from 8 to 15 with there being 14 males and 9 females. Eight of these children were from the study previously mentioned with the remaining coming from admissions to the unit since 1975. Four children were judged to have serious psychopathology thus they were not included in the reporting of these results in anticipation that their fantasy productions would differ significantly in quality and give a skewed view not representative of the typical child in renal failure.

Data was obtained within 3 to 6 weeks from time of admission for dialysis. Each child was interviewed at which time a brief history was taken with emphasis being placed on their social, emotional, and familial circumstances. Each child was then administered the Rorschach and 13 pictures of the Thematic Apperception Test (TAT cards 1, 2, 3 BM, 18 GF, 6 BM, 12 M, 3 GF, 13 MF, 10, 8 BM, 12 F, 16, and 15). Standard instructions for taking each instrument were given. The children were also asked to state three wishes for themselves and an explanation for having given each wish, and they were asked to provide an ending to a story involving an animal family with one of the family members having an illness.

RESULTS AND DISCUSSIONS

Elicited fantasy themes were constricted and surprisingly consistent for all children. The dialyzing child's themes were imbued with fear, aggression, and defense. Aggression was most notably found in stories and productions involving punishment for wrongdoing. In productions of the animal family with a sick member, the children related stories in which a child was sick, and was so because he had been "mean and ugly" or had not obeyed his parents. The TAT produced stories of physical violence and mischief; "She's done something bad. She went with bad girls." This finding is interesting in that it mirrors the formulation of the theory that states that death is viewed as punishment for aggressive impulses.[5,6] Fear and aggression themes contained content that dealt with illness in its broad sense, and also in the specific sense of being sick or the desire to avoid illness or harm. On both the TAT and Rorschach there was mention of missing, broken, or mutilated objects or body parts, for example: "He might be trapped in a mine and might have been in an explosion and lost his arms." The number of anatomy responses on the Rorschach was over twice that which is expected to occur in this population age group.[7] The link between aggression, punishment, and illness would seem to point toward a perception by the child of his health problems being the result of punishment for some act he may have committed.

Not surprisingly, the elicited fantasy productions presented a picture of the world being seen as confusing, hostile, threatening, and fearful. Time and again the indication was that the environment was foreboding, uncertain, and unpredictable. Additionally, it was viewed with mistrust and suspiciousness.

The theme of dependency was also prevalent though not quite as frequent in its appearance as that of the fear and aggression theme. Specifically, the dependency theme was expressed through cooperative efforts involving play, aiding and peaceful efforts, and otherwise drawing others into a helping posture. The content of the dependency theme often portrayed two people building an object or a person caring for an animal. A most interesting finding was that themes involving dependency and cooperativeness almost always had as their main characters humans, who, by the way, were adults, which is contrasted to the themes involving fear and aggression that had as their major characters animals. The interpretation and significance of coupling dependency with adult cooperative efforts is apparent. The attachment and dependency literature[8,9] repeatedly has demonstrated the importance of the attachment figure's accessibility and predictability, particularly during high-stress periods, for the reduction of anxiety and increased security in the child.

It is suggested that the preponderance of the two major fantasy themes—that is, fear–aggression and dependency—as the two major conflicting areas in the child's life are operating in concert to assure stability of adjustment. Fantasy themes not only reflect the negative incentives they wish to avoid but also the positive incentives for which they strive. When in conflict, as when life is threatened or separation from the world seems possible, those in greatest conflict may entertain fear themes in fantasy. Juxtaposed to this phenomenon is the apparent fact that the children avoid acting out these fantasy themes in their overt behavior with the intensity and nakedness they had experienced in fantasy. It would appear that there is a direct inverse correlation between the child's fantasies and his typical patterns of overt behavior.

Of the 27 subjects from which data was originally obtained for this study, only four, as mentioned, had behavior that was thought to reflect significant psychopathology. What appears of significance is the fact that the children's overt behavior showed only minimal to moderate degrees of anxiety, the sources of which could not be adequately assessed through a verbal interview. However, efforts to tap their private thoughts led to results that indicated the vast majority of these inner thoughts dealt with such conflict-laden themes as hostile and foreboding environments, suspiciousness and mistrust, and a preoccupation with emotional support and security. Again, of particular note was the intensity and frequency with which these themes tended to reoccur in the child's productions. We see then a curious mixture of overt behavior and fantasy— behavior which gives only little evidence of what seems to be occurring with great and intense occasion in the child's private world. It is suggested that the fantasies of these children serve as a control function by binding the energy associated with their affective states. This binding of energy then serves to regulate and modify the expression of the state. It would thus appear likely that the fantasy thoughts of the children have problem-solving properties that enable these children to make adaptations to very real and life-threatening circumstances.

In viewing the withdrawn versus the engaging groups of children in terms of their use of fantasy themes, no discernable difference was noted in the frequency of the productions of the themes. The withdrawn children tended to produce the dependency theme more frequently than did the engaging children. There was only slight difference in the frequency with which the fear–aggression themes were produced, with the withdrawn group having fewer. The withdrawn children tended to emphasize mistrust and suspiciousness more in the content of their productions which may well help to explain their lack of interaction with those about them. Further, the withdrawn group tended to have fewer productions which were of a shorter length than did the engaging children. The results of the two groups are viewed as consistent and as a substantiation of the conclusions of this study.

CONCLUSIONS

It is concluded that elicited fantasy productions of children in end-stage renal disease can provide valuable information for understanding the psychological state of the child at the time of institution of dialysis. The forms fantasy takes in these children is highly constricted. For the most part, themes of fear, aggression, and dependency are produced suggesting a preoccupation so complete that other more typical childhood fantasies are rare. These fantasies represent conflictual elements in the child's life but are believed to be functioning in concert, much like polar opposites, to assure stability of adjustment. The results also suggest a problem-solving property interpretation of fantasy.

REFERENCES

1. EPSTEIN, S. Toward a unified theory of anxiety. In B. A. Maher (Ed.), *Progress in experimental personality research*, Vol. 4. New York: Academic, 1967, pp. 1–39.
2. SAMPSON, T. F. The child in renal failure; emotional impact of treatment on the child and his family. *Journal of Child Psychiatry*, 1975, 14, 462–476.
3. GUILFORD, J. P. *The Nature of Human Intelligence.* New York: McGraw-Hill, 1967.
4. SINGER, J. L., and ANTROBUS, J. S. A factor-analytic study of day dreaming and conceptually related cognitive and personality variables. *Perceptual and Motor Skills*, 1963, 17, 187–209.
5. ROSENZWEIG, S., and BRAY, D. Sibling death in the awareness of schizophrenic patients. *Archives of Neurology and Psychiatry*, 1943, 49, 71–92.
6. ANTHONY, S. *The child's discovery of death.* London: Kegan Paul, 1940.
7. AMES, L. B., METRAUX, R. W., and WALKER, R. N. *Adolescent Rorschach responses.* New York: Basic Books, 1969.
8. BOWLBY, J. Attachment and loss. *Attachment.* Vol. 1. London, Hogarth; New York: Basic Books, 1969.
9. AINSWORTH, M. D. S. *Infancy in Uganda; infant care and the growth attachment.* Baltimore, Maryland: The Johns Hopkins Press, 1967.

III
Renal Transplantation

18

Psychological Factors Affecting Acceptance or Rejection of Kidney Transplants

JORGE STEINBERG, NORMAN B. LEVY, AND
ANDREAS RADVILA

The Downstate Medical Center has had continuing interest in behavioral observations of patients with end-stage renal disease.[1] With the development of an active renal transplant program here four years ago, members of the Medical Psychiatric Liaison Service extended their activity to the study of the issues facing both transplant recipients and donors. Initially, we met regularly to listen to and to discuss the tape-recorded interviews that one of us (J.S.) had with these patients. From these weekly meetings, a more formal study ensued in which we addressed ourselves to investigating several issues: How do recipients and donors perceive the transplanted organ? What are the major stresses facing these patients? Do psychological factors affect the success or failure of renal transplantation?

In turning to reports about these issues, although a book[2] and about 50 papers on these issues have been published, we were impressed by the paucity of systematic observational data. Concerning the phenomenon of psychological factors affecting organ rejection, Viederman reported a case in which essentially the "giving-up given-up complex" was incrimi-

JORGE STEINBERG, M.D. • Director, Psychiatric Residency Program; and Associate Professor of Clinical Psychiatry, State University of New York, Downstate Medical Center, Brooklyn, New York.   NORMAN B. LEVY, M.D. • Professor of Psychiatry, State University of New York, Downstate Medical Center, Brooklyn, New York. Present affiliation: Director, Psychiatric Liaison Service, Westchester County Medical Center, Valhalla, New York; and Coordinator, Liaison Services, Department of Psychiatry, New York Medical College, New York, New York.   ANDREAS RADVILA, M.D. • Fellow, Psychosomatic Medicine; and Clinical Instructor of Medicine, State University of New York, Downstate Medical Center, Brooklyn, New York. Present affiliation: Department of Medicine, University of Bern, Bern, Switzerland.

nated as the psychological reason for a physiological rejection.[3] Eisendrath reported that 8 out of 11 patients who died following renal transplantations were noted to have a sense of abandonment by the family or to have experienced panic and a sense of pessimism about the outcome of their operation to a degree not observed among patients who survived the procedure.[4] One of the most significant studies on the psychological effects of kidney transplants was conducted by Basch who interviewed recipients of 9 related and 19 cadaveric kidney transplants over a four-year period.[5] He found that family conflicts in the related recipients were heightened by transplantation. Recipients of cadaveric kidneys seemed to be affected by the fantasies about the cadaver and their attitudes toward death and dying. Castelnuovo-Tedesco described the patient's need to cope with an altered body image as playing a significant role in the occurrence of postoperative emotional disturbances.[6] In a study of 12 donors, Fellner and Marshall pointed to the "irrationality" of the usually rapidly made decision to donate a kidney.[7] Their early findings of self-satisfaction and increased self-image of donors of successfully transplanted kidneys were confirmed in the recently reported nine-year follow-up of these subjects.[8] In those transplant donors whose kidneys were eventually rejected, they retrospectively found that they had much ambivalence about their donations. Simmons and Bernstein report on positive effects, namely upon the self esteem of donors of kidneys.[9,10] However, to the best of our knowledge, no investigator has addressed the issue of dynamic and unconscious factors involved in either the decision to donate a kidney or the outcome of transplantation.

METHODS

Throughout 1976 all 26 patients and their donors who were to receive a kidney from a live donor at this medical center were interviewed, usually one day prior to their surgery. All but one recipient were on hemodialysis awaiting a transplant, or were on maintenance hemodialysis as their definitive treatment and were dissatisfied with the quality of life that they had been experiencing. In both groups, hemodialysis was uniformly seen as not able to produce the state of health which they both wanted and thought feasible as a result of receiving a transplant. The high motivation for this procedure alerted us to the fact that a selective process had already taken place in choosing these patients for transplantation. The tape-recorded interviews lasted from 50 minutes to an hour-and-a-half. Subsequent interviews, usually less formally conducted and at bedside, were done about a week after surgery. We were interested in learning how each recipient adapted to end-stage renal disease and hemodialysis, what his expectations for transplantation were, the degree to which he was informed of the possible complications of having an organ transplant, and his knowledge of the effects of immuno-suppressive medications. In addition to learning about each patient's general life-style and psychological symptoms, in the interview we focused on the affective state of each patient, and his object relations, particularly his relationship with the donor.

Concerning donors, in addition to assessing psychological phenomena, their major affects, their life-styles, and their object relations, we focused upon their relationship with the recipients, how it came about that they served as a donor, and the expectations they had from surgery both for themselves and for the recipient.

Following these interviews we met as a study group to discuss our findings. The group consisted of two of us (J.S. and N.B.L.) together with Dr. Anthony Villamena, a Fellow on our service who left this medical center at the end of June, 1976, and was replaced by the junior author of this paper. In our meetings, the data of the separate, recorded interviews of the recipient and of the donor were presented and discussed. We engaged in a predictive study in which we assessed the overall success or failure of the procedure based solely upon psychological factors. The basis of positive evaluations of recipients for success of the procedure was the relative absence of ambivalence toward the procedure and about the donor, realistic expectations about the future, reasonable optimism about the oncoming operative procedure, and a relative lack of serious depressive symptoms. Each of the three of us independently rated the recipients prior to surgery on a scale of 1 to 5, in which those we thought highly unlikely to retain their grafts were rated "1," those unlikely were rated "2," those possible were rated "3," those likely "4," and those very likely to successfully retain the transplanted organ rated "5."

All but 1 of the 26 recipients (Table 1 patient No. 17) received a kidney from live related donations. The recipients were equally divided between men and women. Their mean age was 29.0 years; 15 were white, 8 of Hispanic background, and 3 black. The occupations were: 8 housewives, 7 unemployed, 5 students, 2 secretaries, 2 professionals, 1 unskilled worker, and 1 business person. Sixteen had chronic glomerulonephritis, a classification including renal failure of unknown origin, 2 pyelonephritis, 2 hypertension, 2 lupus erythematosus, 1 diabetes mellitus, 2 gout, and 1 heroin nephropathy. The duration of renal disease ranged from 1 to 12 years and the period of time on hemodialysis from 2 months to 9 years, except for one patient who had never been on hemodialysis. At the time that this report was written, 19 months after the initial patient was seen and 12 months after the last patient in the series was transplanted, there have been three deaths. There were five other patients in whom rejection phenomena made it necessary for the transplanted organ to be removed.

TABLE 1
Donors and Recipients

No.	Recipient	Age	Sex	Donor	Age	Sex	Rejection (R) or death (D)
1	A.Z.	30	F	T.A.	52	M	
2	U.I.	37	M	N.O.	30	F	
3	L.T.	31	M	O.T.	26	M	R
4	C.A.	26	F	R.O.	42	F	R
5	A.U.	40	M	G.I.	37	F	D
6	O.P.	39	F	F.A.	62	F	
7	A.N.	31	M	O.B.	52	F	
8	M.I.	33	F	N.O.	31	F	
9	T.W.	29	F	H.O.	61	F	D
10	C.A.	27	F	N.A.	21	F	D
11	N.S.	18	M	G.S.	19	M	
12	L.T.	27	F	N.M.	50	F	
13	L.E.	24	M	E.E.	53	F	
14	R.M.	31	M	A.D.	30	F	R
15	Y.C.	22	F	A.C.	18	F	
16	E.G.	22	M	A.G.	18	M	
17	D.D.	24	F	R.E.	44	M	R
18	J.F.	37	M	M.T.	70	M	
19	E.V.	18	F	J.V.	46	M	
20	E.H.	15	M	R.H.	53	M	
21	S.R.	27	M	A.R.	49	F	
22	A.F.	30	F	R.F.	49	F	R
23	R.L.	25	M	N.L.	52	F	
24	C.B.	46	F	T.B.	34	F	
25	E.V.	50	M	R.V.	49	M	
26	T.W.	15	M	N.W.	17	M	

The donors, 15 women and 11 men, had a mean age of 41 years. Sixteen donor–recipient pairs were of the same sex and 10 of different sexes. Table 2 shows the relationship between pairs and the numbers in each group. Eleven of the donors were housewives, 4 students, 3 unskilled workers, 2 secretaries, 2 unemployed, 1 business person, 1 professional, 1 skilled worker, and 1 donor's occupation was unknown.

RESULTS

In our predictions as to the success of the transplanted organ, based on psychological data alone, on a scale of 1 to 5, most of our predications were either 3 (possible) or 4 (likely). No patient was rated 1 (highly unlikely) or 5 (very likely). Only in one instance did we give a patient a

TABLE 2
Relationship between Recipients and Donors[a]

Different sex			Same sex		
Son–mother	4	(0)	Sister–sister	5	(1)
Daughter–father	2	(0)	Brother–brother	5	(1)
Brother–sister	1	(1)	Daughter–mother	4	(2)
Sister–brother	1	(1)	Son–father	2	(0)
Niece–aunt	1	(1)	Total	16	(4)
Unrelated	1	(1)			
Total	10	(4)			

[a] Numbers of rejectors in parentheses.

rating of 2 (unlikely). In that case the recipient of the organ was a 26-year-old single teacher who, in earlier years had been very close to her "spinster" aunt who was 22 years her senior. However, the younger woman had broken off the relationship six years before because of the feeling that her aunt was too controlling and did not let her grow up. When the opportunity for transplantation arose, the younger woman's parents and aunt saw this operation as an opportunity to bring the two together again. However, after making the commitment to the donation, the aunt discovered that her niece continued to maintain the same distance from her. Upon being interviewed, the aunt reported telling the recipient, "Take my fucking kidney and I don't want to see you again." As we had predicted, the organ rejected shortly after transplantation.

The mean rating of those 18 patients who retained their kidney was 3.53 and of those 8 who rejected their kidney 3.45, essentially no difference at all. In those 16 pairs of the same sex, there were four rejections and in the 10 of different sexes four rejections. As seen in Table 2, there was no connection between the nature of the relationship between the pairs and the rejection of kidneys.

We found that most recipients had been informed at the onset of their end-stage renal disease that their definitive treatment was a kidney transplant. In general we were impressed by a lack of realistic expectations on the part of most of the patients. When initially interviewed all the recipients had an outlook at least somewhat more positive than transplantation could realistically offer them, an understandable distortion at a time so close to their operation. However, in the case of 13, or half of these patients, there were major disparities between reality and their expectations. Six had no accurate concept of the immunosuppressive medicines or minimized it greatly; seven had no accurate concept of the phenomenon of rejection, although all had been at least informed of its existence.

An ubiquitous wish-fulfilling fantasy held by both donors and recipients was that transplantation would entirely cure the recipients and return them to the way they were before the onset of kidney disease. Such a thought was overtly conscious and verbalized in the two patients with lupus, a systemic life-threatening illness.

In terms of object relations, almost all donors wanted to restore the distance or closeness they had had with the recipients prior to their kidney disease. There were a few exceptions to this, namely where relationships had not been affected by the recipient's kidney disease, or where the donation was seen by the donor as an opportunity to get closer, in fact to merge with the recipient. For example, in the case of patient No. 10, the donor, an unmarried younger woman, said of her gift to her sister, a person whom she admired and envied, "If she has children they will be half mine." In another instance, a brother and sister had been raised by a sadistic father after the death of their mother. In early adulthood the brother had developed kidney disease. His sister viewed her giving her kidney as a way of creating a rebirth of her brother who, in fantasy, would be her son, while she would be their missed mother.

Those donors who were the mothers of the recipients often saw their donation as an opportunity to have a rebirth of their child as a healthy individual. As in other relationships, the usual wish was to reinstate that which existed before illness. In another case a mother donating to her son wished to reestablish the distance she was able to have before he became sick. His illness caused him to rely heavily upon her, necessitating her leaving a comfortable life she had made for herself in a neighboring state in order to nurse him. Her wish was that the successful transplant would enable a reestablishment of the distance she wanted to retain. In another case, an older brother donated his kidney hoping that his sibling would regain his independence and not demand so much from him.

We found six recipients to be moderately depressed and the rest mildly depressed. In addition to the recipient we rated as "unlikely" to accept the transplant and who indeed rejected the graft, four others were overtly ambivalent about the procedure.

In general we were impressed by the extent of commitment to the procedure made by both recipients and donors. At times such commitments necessitated their suppressing, repressing, and failing to learn about its shortcomings. This information, if not offered by physicians, other professional staff, and successful transplant patients who were often seen by future recipients, was certainly available for the asking from these people. It is also quite possible that in some patients the wish that transplantation be a definitive cure caused them to repress information which contradicted the wish.

With the exception of three donors who were directly asked for their kidneys by the future recipients, all donors spontaneously volunteered to donate their organs. This generosity seemed to be based on unconscious guilt, which surfaced usually in terms of feelings about being healthier and having a greater life expectancy than their related recipient. Mother donors wanted a reborn child, probably to expiate the guilt of having given birth to a "defective" one.

Examination of the immunological data, as seen in Table 3, revealed that in our sample of 26 patients in which there were eight rejections, there was no significance between immunological matching with HLA and mixed lymphocyte culture (MLC) responses on the one hand and rejection or acceptance of the organ on the other.

DISCUSSION

We were initially somewhat surprised to find that the accuracy of our predictions of the success or failure of transplantations, based only on psychological factors, was not substantiated by the outcome. However, we need not have been surprised since there are many factors which affect the outcome of transplantation. It is difficult to substantiate a single factor as contributory to the outcome unless there are a good number of patients representing an extreme degree of this variable. In our group there was a selective process which eliminated those patients who, on psychosocial grounds, were grossly unsuitable. There was selection and elimination of many patients because the nature of their family and object ties to family members did not permit them to have a live related donor. In addition, the surgical staff eliminated those donors who were overtly ambivalent about their gift giving. Also, selective processes occurred within families and as a result of advice, direction and/or selection by nephrologists and other professional staff. The future course of some of the cases may effect the statistical significance between prediction and outcome.

TABLE 3
Immunological Data

HLA antigen matches	Nonrejectors	Rejectors
0	1	1
1	1	0
2	12	4
3	2	1
4	2	2
MLC[a] responses		
Positive	13	6
Negative	5	2

[a] Mixed lymphocyte culture.

The hypothesis that psychological rejection or acceptance can affect physiological acceptance or rejection is an attractive concept which might have validity. It would seem to us that when the fantasy of recipient and donor match best, physiological acceptance would be favored. An example of the latter is that of a mother donor's wish to have a rebirth of her child and the recipient joining in that fantasy by seeing the transplant as a new life.

Greater clarification is needed as to what psychosocial stress factors affect outcome. Careful screening is needed as to the willingness to give and to receive a kidney. In addition, we believe these patients need to know early in their treatment the facts surrounding the surgical procedure, such as the chances for success or failure including the details of the morbidity of being on immunosuppressive medications and facing an uncertain future. Otherwise, such a patient, faced with the side effects of medication or with rejection, may become seriously depressed and feel that he was not treated honestly by his physician.

Once the commitment is made to transplantation, the educational process is interfered with because of the potential wish fulfillment involved in the operation. Such a disparity between actual knowledge and future experience will aggravate the disappointment patients experience in finding that the procedure is not all that they hoped it to be. As shown in another study on hemodialysis patients,[11] unrealistic expectations can be a formidable stress which may in itself lead to psychological and medical complications. Further research is needed to clarify the nature of the stress facing kidney recipients and donors and the effects of psychological factors in the overall success or failure of this procedure.

ACKNOWLEDGMENTS. The authors wish to acknowledge the help they received from Drs. Ismail Parsa, Samuel Kountz, Khalid Butt, and Franz Reichsman and Mrs. Ruth Groveman.

REFERENCES

1. LEVY, N. B. Psychological studies at the Downstate Medical Center of patients on dialysis. *Medical Clinics of North America*, 1977, 61, 759–769.
2. CASTELNUOVO-TEDESCO, P. (Ed.) *Psychiatric aspects of organ transplantation.* New York: Grune and Stratton, 1971.
3. VIEDERMAN, M. Psychogenic factors in kidney transplant rejection. *American Journal of Psychiatry*, 1975, 132, 957–959.
4. EISENDRATH, R. M. The role of grief and fear in the death of kidney transplant patients. *American Journal of Psychiatry*, 1969, 126, 381–387.
5. BASCH, S. H. The intrapsychic integration of a new organ. A clinical study of kidney transplantation, *Psychoanalytic Quarterly*, 1973, 41, 364–384.

6. CASTELNUOVO-TEDESCO, P. Organ transplant, body image, psychosis. *Psychoanalytic Quarterly*, 1973, *42*, 349–363.
7. FELLNER, C. H., and MARSHALL, J. R. Kidney donors: the myth of informed consent. *American Journal of Psychiatry*, 1970, *126*, 1245–1251.
8. MARSHALL, J. R., and FELLNER, C. H. Kidney donors revisited. *American Journal of Psychiatry*, 1977, *134*, 575–576.
9. SIMMONS, R. G. and SIMMONS, R. L. Organ-transplantation: a societal problem. *Social Problems*, 1971, *19*, 36–57.
10. BERNSTEIN, D. M. After transplantation—the child's emotional reactions. *American Journal of Psychiatry*, 1971, *127*, 1189–1193.
11. REICHSMAN, F., and LEVY, N. B. Problems in adaptation to maintenance hemodialysis a four-year study of 25 patients. *Archives of International Medicine*, 1972, *130*, 859–865.

19

The Life Trajectory of Patients with Long-Term Kidney Transplants

A Pilot Study

MILTON VIEDERMAN

Renal transplantation has moved from the experimental stage to become a well-established therapeutic procedure. Because of its substantial cost in professional time and money, questions have been raised about its justification in the hierarchy of social priorities. Moreover, the stresses which this operation place on the patient and the family are considerable and involve not only the small degree of risk of death and impairment in a related donor, but also physical and emotional suffering which is compounded in circumstances when the transplant fails. Although the immediate impact of transplantation has been well described in the literature, there are no published long-term studies designed to evaluate the quality of life and the nature of adaptation of patients who maintain viable transplants many years after transplantation.

The present study was designed to examine the experience of illness, of hemodialysis, and of transplantation in order to construct a coherent narrative of the patient's life, and to evaluate the degree to which one could determine how these particular experiences influenced it. The study attempts to answer two questions:

1. How effectively can one evaluate the impact of transplantation on patients who have maintained the kidney for over five years? To what degree does the fear of loss of the kidney remain a significant influence? What fantasies about the kidney persist? To what degree is the kidney integrated in the patient's body schema?
2. What factors in the life experiences of these patients and what aspects of their character most influence the answer to the above question?

MILTON VIEDERMAN, M.D. • Professor of Clinical Psychiatry, Cornell University Medical College; and Rogosin Kidney Center, New York Hospital, New York, New York. This was made possible by support from the NIMH Psychiatry Education Branch, Grant MH 14747-04.

The method of this study involved partially structured clinical interviews. Each of four patients was interviewed on audiotape for an hour during four successive weeks.* Though no statistical conclusions can be drawn about the general outcome of transplantation based upon a sample of four patients, the pilot project has been useful. Although one could arrive at some reasonably confident conclusions about the quality of the patient's life at a moment in time, earlier influences on the current state are not always as easy to trace and to convincingly demonstrate. Hence, it was not surprising that the experience of transplantation often became interwoven in the fabric of the patient's experience and could not be seen as a discrete event having an unambiguous influence on the present.

However, the intensive interview experience was a useful method of determining which experiences in the past most effected the current situation. The richness of the material permitted inferences about unconscious influences. Spreading the interviews over a period of weeks permitted the patient to become familiar with the interviewer and resulted in each case in greater spontaneity and opportunity for the patient to reveal his predominant preoccupations. In this light, one of the most interesting aspects of the study was the intensity of what was generated in each patient in the form of transference reactions, insights, demands for reassurance, and interpretation. In one case, the interviews stimulated the dramatic revelations of a family secret. What we had expected to be a situation of relatively neutral observation, became, in essence, a highly demanding brief therapy. The reactions of the patients became important sources of data about their character and their perception and interaction with the world.

This initial project will be followed by a systematic study of all of the more than 40 patients at the Rogosin Kidney Center who have had transplants for more than five years. The subsequent study will complement the interviews with a battery of psychological tests which will include general scales related to adaptation, depression, and anxiety, as well as cognitive scales, projective tests, and figure drawings.

After a brief review of the relevant literature, the case histories will be described in considerable detail so as to permit a discussion of the individual character of each patient's adaptation and response to the illness and treatment. A brief statement about the impact of the study on the individual patients will be made. Transference reactions will be described, though it is recognized that given the limited nature of the contact, much of this remains inferential. This will be followed by a discussion of the questions posed at the beginning of the paper (refer to Table 1 for an outline of case histories).

*I would like to express my appreciation to Dr. Andrea Clair, who performed the interviews and discussed them with me.

There are no completed studies of a large group of patients who have had transplants for at least five years. Simmons, Klein, and Simmons have recently completed a one year posttransplant follow-up of 156 patients.[1] They used quantitative scales to measure the patient's perceived level of physical rehabilitation, his general psychosocial adjustment, and his ability to perform in occupational and school roles. In almost all of these categories, the patient showed a dramatic improvement compared to their pretransplant level of adaptation. Even diabetics who were initially more impaired, showed significant improvement. The authors comment on the maintenance of the "sick role" in some patients as well as the presence of societal barriers to vocational rehabilitation, in particular, difficulties in obtaining health insurance. (Patient No. 2 illustrates these problems.) They comment also on the fact that certain groups are more likely to present problems in adaptation and include the following: adolescents, men rather than women, persons of low income and education, individuals who show less favorable adjustment pretransplant, patients whose appearance has been very negatively effected by their steroid medication, and individuals who receive less emotional support from the family.

Muslin is in the process of completing a long-term follow-up of patients with kidney transplants.[2] He finds that a substantial number of his patients have only a modest to moderate enhancement of the quality of their lives, and that this seems to be related to the degree to which the kidney has been internalized as part of the body schema. In previous work, he outlined the phases of internalization of the kidney, a process which he feels is not completed in many patients.[3,4] He outlines three phases: (1) the foreign body stage, (2) the stage of partial internalization, and (3) the stage of complete internalization. He emphasizes that external stimuli may evoke a regression to a foreign body reaction (as was observed in Patient No. 2).

Beard described in detail the posttransplantation experience of five patients.[5] Only two of his patients had had their transplants for as long as nine months, and these were the only patients who showed reliable indications of a significant improvement in the quality of their lives. The other patients, who were only six months posttransplant, revealed much anxiety and "ambivalent conflicts between fear and hope, dependence and independence, apathy and involvement. . . ." Abram found that 30 patients who had transplants ranging from five years to less than a year were doing remarkably well.[6] Similarly, George reported that 35 transplant patients from 10 to 24 months after surgery had a very high percentage of return to employment or housework.[7] Eisendrath underlines the extreme vulnerability of posttransplant patients to object loss and found that of 11 patients who died following kidney transplantation, nine had complications which had a temporal relationship to loss of significant objects.[8]

The extensive literature on the integration of the organ into the body schema, and the dynamics of the difficulties which ensue will not be discussed.[2–4,7,9–14]

CASE HISTORIES

Refer to Table 1 for an outline of the case histories.

Patient No. 1: Mr. G

Mr. G is a 30-year-old divorced bank clerk, who leads a rich and active life 5½ years after transplantation.

In the interview situation and elsewhere the patient used helplessness to evoke positive responses from people and was able to elicit support regularly from friends because of his warmth and general appeal. There was little depression and he experienced considerable pleasure in life.

Mr. G was noted to have albumin in his urine during adolescence. He was 22 and working at a bank when renal failure became severe enough to necessitate dialysis. After 2½ years of home dialysis, during which he continued to work, he received a transplant which he has had for 5½ years. There have been no substantial rejection episodes. Moderate complications of Prednisone treatment have resulted in glaucoma, muscle pain, and weakness.

Early History

The patient was born to a lower middle class family. Father was described as an aggressive, highly critical man, who thoroughly intimidated the patient. Mother was seen as a hypochondriacal, passive, frightened woman, who was often sick. She was highly overprotective, would overdress her son, and constantly required him to report his whereabouts to her. Mother died when the patient was 10 of cancer of the uterus which was diagnosed only a few days before her death. One year later, the father married a strong, firm, affectionate woman, who encouraged independence, was not overprotective, though she was somewhat controlled. The patient maintains a good relationship with her.

Mr. G's memories of his childhood are reasonably happy ones. Though he viewed himself as a sickly child and was poor at athletics, he had many friends and did average school work. He had two years of junior college before he returned to live at home and begin work.

The Impact of Illness and Transplantation

When, at the age of 22, the patient was informed that he had terminal renal failure and required dialysis, he responded with panic and tears. Only when his stepmother intervened and took over did he feel reassured. She controlled the home dialysis entirely and insisted that no matter how he felt, he had to remain on the machine for a full eight-hour period. Often he was symptomatic with cramps, headaches, nausea, and vomiting. However, between periods of dialysis, he systematically kept the thoughts of dialysis out of his mind. He worked, experienced considerable pleasure in life, and felt very supported by his friends and family who "were living the experience with me."

The offer of a cadaver kidney when he was 24 evoked panic and a need to seek reassurance from his stepmother with whose support he accepted the operation. The day that the kidney began to work, he felt that it was his, but there was considerable anxiety about possible rejection during the first six months after the transplantation. This has gradually subsided, and he is not currently troubled with anxiety about rejection, though he is aware of the possibility that it may occur. There is a lingering avoidance of the *NAPHT Journal* for fear of seeing articles which describe rejection in long-term transplantation patients. To return to dialysis would be a terrible diasppointment, but the patient feels that he could tolerate it. Though the patient jokes about taking on some of the characteristics of the cadaver donor, he has successfully integrated the kidney in his body schema and does not experience it as a foreign body.

Since his transplantation, Mr. G has undergone a number of life changes, which reflect maturation. In the context of a brief therapy which began a year ago, he has begun to sail, ski, bike, and generally engage in athletic activities. This is new to him and striking in the light of his view of himself as particularly clumsy and unathletic as a child. In these activities, he is appropriately, but not excessively, cautious, and there is little to suggest a counterphobic motivation. On the few occasions when he received a blow to the abdomen around the site of the transplanted kidney, he responded appropriately and without excessive anxiety.

Two years ago, the patient married a strong, independent woman, whom he saw as the "ideal mate." He married her with the realization that he would need a woman to take care of him if ever he were sick again. His wife had been aware of the fact that he had been on dialysis, that he had had a transplant, and that there was a possibility that dialysis might again be necessary. Particularly important to him was her interest in his illness and treatment. She is described in a way strongly reminiscent of the stepmother. One year after the marriage, his wife became disenchanted with the patient's excessive attachment to his family, some of his childlike qualities, and requested separation and divorce. Though he was initially quite depressed, he has tolerated the separation quite well and would like to marry again. It is worthy of note that in spite of his vulnerability to loss, this experience did not have somatic repercussions.

Current Adaptation

The patient has had steady promotions at work, where his professional goals seem consonant with his ability. He is in the process of completing his bachelor's degree at night. He maintains an active social life, has close friends, and though he experiences conflicts with women, he expects to remarry in the future. Since transplantation, he has maintained an active sexual life, though he does suffer from premature ejaculation. (At no point did he have difficulty in having erections.)

Mr. G continues to live within an eight-block radius of his parents' home

TABLE 1

	Early experience, central conflicts	Adaptation to illness and TP	Transference
Patient #1: Progressive development	Early over-protection by worried mother who died when patient was 10 Stepmother: Affectionate, strong, supportive, controlling	Excellent Illness "in past" Dissolution of inhibitions in physical activity	Wish for direction Sexual attraction Maternal transfer-ence (stepmother)
Patient #2: Regression in face of illness	Early deprivation Early independence Responsibility Care for others "Do not take"	Regressive return of early depriva-tion in absence of job Anger Despair Fall in self-esteem	"I can get nothing" Reevocation of early parental experience Parental trans-ference
Patient #3: Blocked development	Intense sibling rivalry for mother's attention Use of sick role to win attention and to defeat and alienate sister	Utilization to maintain special role in family Bland but comfort-able Not unhappy existence	"Reassure me" Helplessness to obtain support and attention Maternal trans-ference
Patient #4: Grief response of middle adulthood	Rich early life Oedipal attachment to brother leading to inhibition in sustaining special relationship	Relatively good adjustment to illness and TP Crisis of middle adulthood Severe incapacitating cardiac disease	Curative fantasy Wished for idealized good mother

Attitude to physician	Insights	Effects of i.v.
Good relationship	Recognizes: (1) that he handles current Rx as he handled dialysis, "putting out of mind," fearful of dependence on therapist as on machine (2) that his negative self-valuation stems in part from illness	Splitting of transference Confrontation of therapist with dissatisfaction No other evident change
Bitter complaint "They do not care"	Awareness of anger Inability to take	Will seek Rx
Distance Complaints	Awareness of her use of illness Awareness of intimidation of mother	Revelation of family secrets by mother Patient's confrontation with father
Good relationship	Awareness of wish to talk to "good mother"	Catharsis Initiation of previously aborted grief reaction Reworking of past

(interesting in light of the fact that this was the limit his mother imposed on his freedom to wander from home when he was a child). Moreover, he has internalized some of his stepmother's prohibitions—namely, that he be home at 11 p.m. during the week and not after 2 a.m. on weekends.

He experiences little in the way of somatic symptoms. Mild, occasional depression is usually related to some competitive failure. Clearly, Mr. G obtains a great deal of pleasure from life and has hope for the future.

The patient has little anxiety about kidney loss and has in the last five years begun to use his "reclining dialysis chair" something he could not do for the first few years after transplantation.

His return to the Catholic Church after the transplantation was at first a way of "paying back for what had been given me," but now has become a meaningful aspect of his life.

Impact of Study

Mr. G had a positive response to the interviewer whom he saw as giving, supportive, and, by implication, a good mother. These feelings contrasted strongly with the anger which he described toward his psychotherapist, whom he viewed as depriving, nonguiding, and nonsupportive. He did not reveal that he was in psychotherapy until the third session, and it is likely that he was splitting the transference. Dreams of a strange woman to whom he was attracted and an inexplicable sense of depression during the last session, suggested that intense feelings had been generated by the interviews.

The patient had a number of insights during the interview. He realized that he was isolating the current psychotherapy from the rest of his life in a way which was reminiscent of the way he handled his hemodialysis. This reflected his need to avoid recognition of dependence both upon the therapist and on the dialysis machine. The similarity between his dependence on his former wife and his dependence upon his stepmother also became apparent to him.

The interviews acted as a stimulus in his own therapy where he began to examine more clearly his negative feelings toward his therapist which had been highlighted by the contrasting attitude toward the interviewer.

Comment and Formulation

Mr. G has done extremely well in spite of a significant potential for regressive incapacitation based upon an identification with a doting, over-protective mother who was also hypochondriacal, anxious, and worrying. This tendency would have been accentuated by the mother's sudden death when the patient was 10 had it not been for her rapid replacement by a stepmother who was strong and caring, and consistently encouraged growth and independence despite her tendency to control. This encouragement of independence and maturity represents an ideal toward which the patient continues to strive, in the face of strong wishes to depend upon his parents and on his psychotherapist who frustrates this wish.

In light of his early experience with his mother, one might easily have expected that the patient would be given to hypochondriacal reactions, to somatization, or to a disabling anxiety about a possible rejection of the kidney. Though clearly still caught in the conflict between the wish to be dependent and the wish to care for himself, his illness has not been used for this purpose.

Patient No. 2: Mr. I

Mr. I is a 48-year-old married father of two adopted children who has had a transplant for six years.

The patient prided himself on his success as a tug boat captain until his illness ten years ago but has not worked since. He presented himself as an embittered, grudgingly compliant, defeated, resigned, and disabled shadow of a man. He angrily complained of the indifference of the world and particularly of the doctors. He viewed himself as a "have not" dominated by those who have position and material comfort. He reveals marked distress; he sleeps poorly, lacks energy and initiative, and wonders whether it would have been better to die. There is a great deal of guilt about his not having provided properly for his family. Most striking is his description of the dramatic change in his personality which occurred when he became ill, and his sense of betrayal when the transplant did not make him the man he had been.

When the patient was 20, he received a medical discharge from the Army when albumin was noted in his urine. Increasing problems with hypertension, fatigue, and headaches led to hospitalization in his early 30's, and he began dialysis when he was 36. He was on dialysis for four years, three of them at home, and then received a cadaver transplant six years ago. Though he has no significant rejection episodes, there have been complications of Prednisone treatment, including muscle weakness and thrombophlebitis. Though he regards himself as physically debilitated, his limitations are predominantly psychological.

Early History

The patient was born to a lower class family and was the middle child of five brothers and one sister. There is much suppression and repression with rationalization as he describes his early life of marked deprivation. "There is no point in digging up old graves, you're not going to seek vengeance or anything." "We don't remember much—what does a kid remember?"

Mother was an alcoholic about whom he remembers little. He had no contact with her after his parents were separated when he was six years old. The court assigned custody of the children to the father. Father worked at two jobs and was rarely home. He emphasizes his early self-reliance and the control which the children maintained over themselves, their emotions, and their lives. A brother, two years his senior, is an idealized and powerful figure who "looked out for him."

The patient left school to work at a number of jobs, each time rapidly advancing until he began to work on a tug boat which he loved. At 22, he married his first girlfriend, who has remained a supportive responsive wife, tolerant of his irascible nature. Because his wife was unable to conceive, they adopted two children. He advanced rapidly in his work and became a captain in his late 20s. Though this was a heavy responsibility with which he was never entirely comfortable, he continued at this work until he became ill.

These were very happy years for the patient. He describes a devil-may-care attitude, emphasizing his freedom from anxiety, his activity, independence, self-reliance, and particularly his satisfaction at being the undisputed provider for his family. He describes himself as a "go-getter and a self-motivated self-starter." Characteristically, he was reluctant to take from anyone.

He insisted that his wife give up her job. Clearly, this man had a great deal of self-respect during this period, based upon responsibility, productive work, and most important, the feeling that he was giving to his family that which he had never received.

Adaptation to Illness and Current Adaptation

Until the patient became ill, he manifested marked denial and isolation of feeling with regard to the impending deterioration of his kidneys about which he had been informed years before. The impact of illness struck him when he could no longer maintain his activity in work because of increasing fatigue and swelling of the legs. He was very uremic at this time and speaks bitterly about the difficulties of arranging for dialysis which was accomplished through the intervention of his older brother who, in his view, rescued him.

The patient's adaptation to dialysis was poor. He had many symptoms while on dialysis and felt like a prisoner whose life was regulated by a machine. His dependence upon other people was very troublesome. He was told by a physician that his impotence was a physiological response to dialysis, though he was able to have nocturnal erections. After obtaining a job as a long-distance truck driver, he was dissuaded from this activity by a physician because of the threat to his shunt.

The patient was particularly embittered when he received a transplant six years ago and realized that it did not effect the changes in him which he had expected. He never regained his self-confidence, his initiative, his cheerful hopefulness, and he was affected particularly by his failure to provide for his family.

His attitude toward most physicians and toward the social system is a prototype and an expression of his general dissatisfaction with the world. He describes physicians as concerned only with his clinical state and quite indifferent to his feelings, unwilling to answer questions or to treat him with respect. He spontaneously engaged in a repetitive and stereotyped litany against the physicians and the social system. "Only those with money can get what they need to rebuild a productive life after transplantation." His one effort after the transplantation to obtain a job in government service came to naught when he discovered that he would lose his medicare during a two-year probationary period at the job.

The patient is aware of the fact that his kidney came from a 15-year-old who died in a fire. His impulse to express gratitude was inhibited by a sense that he could not approach the family since he had not returned to work. He felt ashamed and unworthy of the gift. To take from others engenders guilt and a need to repay. This is exemplified also by his unwillingness to have considered a living related donor. His wife commented to him that although he refused to take things from his brother on a number of occasions, he expressed great bitterness when they were given to someone else. He was highly critical of a patient in the bed next to him, who was suicidal after having received a transplant from his brother. The patient felt that he should have killed himself before, if this was his intent. Clearly, to take something from someone limited one's freedom and autonomy. In spite of this, the thought of losing the kidney was not an important preoccupation, and there was no evidence that he was overprotective of it.

The dramatic turnabout of this man's view of himself which took place at the time he became ill has had repercussions in all areas of his life. He is a misanthrope, isolated from everyone but his immediate family, and, even in this situation, is irritable, dissatisfied, perfectionistic, and controlling. He appreciates his wife's forebearance, support, and "tolerance" but feels that he has let her down.

Some months following the interviews, the patient was hospitalized for a serious leg ulcer. The physicians discussed the possibility of diminishing the dose of Prednisone which would increase the risk to the kidney. He indicated that he would rather lose the leg than the kidney. He stated: "It has been good to me. It has kept me alive while my children were growing up." The patient thereby expressed his sense of obligation to this personified organ. The threat of loss reevoked the sense of obligation which was related to this man's characterological attitude toward taking.

Impact of Study

The bitterness and anger which the patient experienced toward the world was also directed toward the interviewer. He engaged in a repetitious litany of how badly the world and the medical profession had treated him. He became irritated at the interviewer at any point when she seemed to interfere with this control or challenged him in ways which appeared to him to be condescending. He reiterated that he would be disappointed by the "program," though it had been pointed out to him that there was no primary therapeutic intent in the research plan. He disparaged supportive comments. The interviewer was cast in the role of the depriving mother.

In spite of these complaints, the patient revealed that he had spoken to the interviewer about things he had never mentioned before. This particularly pertained to doubts about whether his current existence was worthwhile and whether it wouldn't be preferable to die. He was particularly struck by his defeatist attitude as he heard himself talk and revealed that he had been ruminating for some time about seeking psychiatric help. He rejected the interviewer's encouragement in this direction until she interpreted his general reluctance to take from anyone. At this point, his tone changed, he confirmed this interpretation with a number of examples and indicated that he would seriously consider psychiatric referral.

Comment and Formulation

The patient had successfully coped with early emotional deprivation by becoming independent, self-reliant, and by not taking from others. His success in life before illness was quite admirable, but it is clear that his self-confidence and self-esteem were contingent upon his working at a responsible job and particularly in caring for himself, his wife, and the children, as *he* had not been cared for. He was unable to cope with the requirements which illness imposed upon him—namely, that of depending upon a machine and on other persons without serious damage to his self-esteem and sense of masculinity. The transplantation was unsuccessful in providing a magical rescue from this predicament, predominantly because he was unable to work out a personally valued and socially acceptable situation after maximum physical recovery. His efforts to find a job were frustrated by external circumstance. One can only speculate about whether success in helping this patient to find a meaningful job might have solidified his self-esteem, diminished his depression, and decreased his sense of futility. The treatment of the depression itself might have changed his life. His previous adaptation would suggest that this might be the case.

This man's bitter complaint about the failure of society and the physicians to rehabilitate him reflect, in important measure, a reevocation of his early sense of maternal deprivation and a rationalization of this in terms of societal failure.

This patient is an example of psychological invalidism after transplantation.

Patient No. 3: Mrs. D

Mrs. D is a 33-year-old married, childless, suburban housewife, who had received a transplant seven years before.

The patient is an unspontaneous, bland woman whose soft, timid, and monotonous voice was punctuated by an anxious giggle when she was unsure of the interviewer's reaction to something she said. As she became more comfortable, the theme of a fierce competitive struggle with her sister for the care and attention of her parents emerged. The atmosphere of family intrigue had a childlike quality. There was little depression and the patient was generally satisfied with her life.

Albuminurea was noted and a diagnosis of glomerulonephritis was made at the time the patient was undergoing an operation for a congenital strabismus at the age of seven. Though asymptomatic, she was treated with a number of special diets and "experimental drugs." At the age of 25, four months after her marriage, Mrs. D was placed on hemodialysis for terminal renal failure. After one year on dialysis, she received a transplant from her father and has done well for seven years without medical complications.

Early History

The patient was born to a lower middle class family which included father, mother, and a sister 14 months her junior. Father is described as "a moody, temperamental, unpredictable, and stubborn man." Throughout her childhood and adult life, their mutual "stubbornness" resulted in frequent arguments. The patient particularly resented his open favoritism of the younger sister. Mother is described as a worrier who is less mercurial than the father or the patient. The mother maintained strict "impartiality" in her behavior toward the two girls. Only sickness led to special indulgence from her.

Though highly competitive, the sisters were extremely attached to one another. The younger sister particularly resented the special attention which fell to the patient because of her illness and describes her pleasure at the opportunity to be hospitalized for a tonsillectomy because of the wonderful gifts she would receive. This close relationship was suddenly interrupted when the patient was 21, and her sister became engaged. Mrs. D particularly envied and resented her sister for abandoning her by finding an attractive man and marrying before she did.

The patient summarized her childhood rather blandly as a happy one.

Except for repeated fights with her father, she enjoyed school and had many friends. Illness and hospitalization played an important part in her early life, and although she felt a sense of shame about being different from other people which has persisted, she also remembers the pleasure of receiving special presents and attention from her mother when she was sick. She has internalized the mother's overprotective prohibitions and still hesitates to go to the beach for fear of "catching the famous chill."

The patient completed college, obtained a master's degree, and worked as a professional in a hospital before she became ill. She describes this with the same lack of enthusiasm and blandness which permeates her view of life. Her husband, whom she met when she was 23, is pictured as a "quiet, steady man" who dotes and worries over her as her mother does. The marriage is comfortable but without passion. The patient is not apparently troubled about not having children, though she avoids "child-oriented women."

The Impact of Illness

Until the patient began dialysis at the age of 25, she isolated any feelings of concern about future kidney failure. Hemodialysis, which was begun only four months after her marriage, was difficult for her. She hated the needles and the sight of blood and was fearful that the staff would not succeed in placing the needles, though apparently there were no access problems. "I looked good but felt lousy, and I could never think clearly as I had done in the past." She felt passive and dependent when on dialysis, and it seemed to her that she was "vegetating." Since beginning dialysis, she has not worked.

A family crisis developed when the issue of a related donor transplant was raised. The patient was very fearful of transplantation and reluctant to accept it. Her sister's husband opposed the sister's participation as a potential donor and moved his family to another state so as to avoid the possibility that she might be chosen. The patient is very resentful of this and has not spoken to the sister since this time. Mother and father similarly broke contact with the sister but reestablished a relationship some years later unbeknownst to the patient.

The patient was surprised to discover that her father was a four antigen match and in response to pressure from him and her husband, she decided to accept the kidney. During the first two and a half months, she experienced two rejection episodes, but since discharge, she has been troubled neither by rejection nor by the side effects of the medications.

Current Adaptation

Mrs. D appears to have a comfortable existence though she remains moderately protective of the kidney. She attempts to avoid colds (the internalization of her mother's protectiveness) and is careful during sexual activity so as not to bruise the transplant. Though her worry about the loss of the kidney is not a constant preoccupation, she anticipates that it will always be with her. Her quarterly annual visits to the hospital are regularly associated with a great deal of fear that the doctors will discover something wrong with the kidney. She hates going to the clinic where she sees the machines, and is reminded of a possible return to hemodialysis. Similarly, she avoids other patients. When the patient discovers a minor symptom, she worries but avoids calling the doctor. Although her concern about the loss of the kidney is not pervasive and dominant, it is clear that she has not fully integrated the organ into her body schema. She was puzzled and unsure when asked whether the kidney was hers and then described it as "temperamental and changeable," words she had used to describe her father. When this was pointed out to her, she laughingly replied that she trusted the kidney more than her father.

Most important is the secondary gain which accrued at the time of the transplant. She remembered her long-standing jealousy of her sister because of her father's favoritism. This was accentuated when the sister was married before she was. She recognized that she had had a perverse satisfaction at the sister's rejection by the family and was angry that the parents had surreptitiously been seeing the sister, who four years before had moved back to the general area where they had been living without her knowledge. Also irritating was the mother's revelation to her that she was intimidated because she had been fearful of "upsetting the sick child." Her illness and her transplant had offered a great deal of secondary gain which she still utilized.

Apart from these preoccupations, the patient lives the life of a suburban housewife. There is no financial pressure or personal motivation to return to work. She plays golf and has a circle of personal friends whom she meets regularly. Her marriage is stable, and she readily admits that she never had much sexual passion. Although she might well have had children had she not become sick, she appears not to regret this. Her vacations with her husband are a source of pleasure and one has the sense that her life would not be very much different had she not become sick.

Impact of Study

Though initially hesitant and concerned about the appropriateness and normality of her feelings, the patient gradually became more spontaneous as she spoke of the competitive relationship with her sister and the feelings of abandonment and jealousy which the sister's marriage evoked in her. In the context of this discussion, the patient became aware of the special gain which had accrued to her from the rift in the family which followed the transplantation and particularly the pleasure which she experienced at being the only object of her parents' attention. In addition, she recognized how she used the sick role to intimidate the mother, who was fearful of upsetting her and thereby prevented the mother from being frank with her.

The research had an impact on the family. The mother used the "support" implicit in the psychiatric interviews to permit herself to reveal to the patient that there had been a surreptitious relationship with the previously exiled sister for many years. It was in the context of this increased frankness that the patient expressed her resentment to the father for his favoritism of the sister. She was pleased that for the first time in her life, the father had listened and not argued. The patient had discovered a new assertiveness with him.

Comment and Formulation

This woman has done well after transplantation. The transplant crystallized a partially latent competitive struggle with her sister. The exclusion of the sister from the family resulted in a competitive success which afforded the patient much gratification, though not without some guilt. Nevertheless, she was perfectly content to see her sister excluded from the family and has been quite disturbed to discover that the exclusion had not been total and that contact had been reestablished. In spite of the gratification incumbent upon the "sick role," this role has not been accentuated in her current life. The patient does not experience herself as a sick person, and the limitations which she imposes upon herself are minimal.

One cannot ignore the price which this family paid for the conflict which transplantation evoked. The many years of bitterness and anger which this situation engendered have left a guilty residue in the patient, particularly because of the gratification afforded.

This woman has not fully integrated the kidney into her self concept. The kidney continues to maintain the attributes of the father–donor, i.e., "temperamental and changeable." The threat of rejection, which does worry the patient, reflects a hostile relationship with her father, who has many times rejected her in anger. The kidney retains the quality of a hostile introject seven years after transplantation though the reaction is attenuated.[11,13,14]

Patient No. 4: Mrs. F

Mrs. F is a 50-year-old, twice married, childless woman who lives with her second husband after having immigrated to the United States from Eastern Europe ten years ago. She has had a functioning transplant for seven years.

Although there had been no major rejection episodes, coronary artery disease and a troublesome arrhythmia are responsible for considerable debilitation. The patient spoke English with a heavy Slavic accent. Rich emotionality gave her story a note of drama and tragedy, but it was never maudlin, superficial, or histrionic. There was an epic quality which suggested a novel by Tolstoy. The patient saw herself as strong, sensitive, thoughtful, and introspective. Although at times she was tearful and occasionally depressed, she maintained a sense of humor, and conveyed a sense of pride, courage and a capacity to act to overcome feelings of weakness, and to struggle courageously with life. It was clear that she was now forced to live in moderate circumstances caring for an ailing mother, plagued by ill health, and far away from her native country. This is very different from the privileged world from which she came. The sessions had a quality of a life review in a physically ill woman who was struggling with the conflicts of middle age.

Thirteen years ago during a brief hospitalization for depression after her father's death, it was noted that the patient had albumin in her urine. Nine years before (one year after having migrated to this country), she developed terminal renal failure and, after one-and-a-half years on dialysis, received a transplant. For seven years, this transplant has functioned well, though her arrhythmia is troublesome.

Early Life

The patient comes from a wealthy, cultured, Jewish-Hungarian family, which had a retinue of servants, including a governess. The primary family survived both the Nazi and Russian occupations, though many relatives were lost in the holocaust. Father was considerably older than the mother at the time of their marriage and, though he was extremely strict, strong, and controlling, she adored him. His death in 1965 evoked a brief depression in the patient. Mother was seen as a busy, but superficial, social woman, who had had little contact with the children. The patient feels that her mother never understood her and did little to create a sense of self-confidence. Mother was a practical woman who was insensitive to the patient's romantic inclinations and insisted that one should marry for money. The mother, now infirm and dependent upon the patient, has always been viewed as a helpless, pampered child. The patient's only sibling was an adored brother, two years her junior. She tended to protect him and to mother him, and even after his marriage continued to indulge him by concealing his extramarital affairs from the family. She enjoyed his jealousy of her boyfriends. His death at the age of 30 of uremia was a great shock to the patient. At his request, she took him from the hospital when he was in a terminal state and, unbeknownst to her parents and his wife, nursed him through the night until he died. She encouraged his wife who was pregnant to have the child and offered to raise it as her own. The erotization of this relationship is very apparent.

During the Nazi occupation, the patient was baptized as a Catholic and sent to live in a convent where only the nuns knew that she was Jewish. She has a sense of shame about this concealment which she feels was cowardly and humiliating.

Mrs. F had a number of experiences with men in her late adolescence and early adulthood. As an adolescent, she had a romantic affair with a 24-year-old pilot which ended in pregnancy after what she describes as a quasirape. This pregnancy was aborted. A three-year marriage in her late 20s to a jealous, alcoholic man ended when she left the man and arranged a divorce. Only once did the patient experience a great passion in her life and feel that she was truly in love. In spite of the rich and intense mutuality which she experienced with this man, who was somewhat younger than she (like the brother), they separated after repeated quarrels years later. Six years ago, during a trip to Romania, the patient saw him again and was very reassured to discover that they still loved one another. In the context of her current concerns about a lack of desire for men and a feeling of deadness, she states rather poignantly that she wishes that she could once again return to Romania to find out whether the old feeling still remains.

Attitude Toward Illness and Current Adaptation

In spite of the fact that her brother died of uremia, the patient reacted minimally to the news that she had kidney disease. The advent of terminal renal failure brought with it a severe organic brain syndrome and the delusion that her feces had come from a man. Hemodialysis, itself, posed no major difficulties, although this was a period of adaptation to a new country, where she had to learn a new language and care for a dependent mother. Dialysis seemed a temporary expedient as she awaited transplantation. The transplant was greeted enthusiastically and experienced as a rebirth. Particular pleasure was associated with her ability to pass bloody urine for the first time in over a year. The transplant was like a second life, a return from "the dead." However, the experience was not without guilt. "Sometimes, I think that I haven't been able to straighten out my life after the transplant because I shouldn't be alive, and it's a punishment." The patient had the fantasy of going to the donor's grave with flowers and initially was guilty that someone had to die for her, that this "person who had made her so happy was dead."

A short flurry of anxiety about rejection occurred when her "surgical twin" (the patient who had received a kidney from the same cadaver) rejected the kidney. At this time, she became anxious and made an error in her medication which was potentially self-destructive. Although there is no current anxiety about the kidney, Mrs. F is having serious difficulty with an arrhythmia and has actively solicited the opinion of a cardiologist about the possibility of cardiac surgery. She would be willing to take the risk for the hope of a better life.

The patient has not worked since her arrival in this country. She states that she would happily work were it not for her arrhythmia and the obligation to care for her mother. She remains active: embroidering, decorating, and redecorating her house which she calls her "beautiful prison." Though there are times when she awakens with little energy, little desire to do things, she forces herself to engage in work and is able to overcome this inertia and depression. The patient is currently married to a man she has known since her early twenties. Though highly successful in his old country, he has essentially given up here and is satisfied with a menial job which is far below his training and capacity. She feels that their roles are reversed, that she has to remain strong and to mother him. The relationship lacks a sense of intimacy.

Impact of Study

The patient was spontaneous and gave the impression throughout the interviews of engaging in a thoughtful life review. She cried a great deal both during and in between sessions, behavior which was quite uncharacteristic of her. The sadness and grief which she displayed as she talked about her life suggested a mourning process and had the quality of a catharsis. She seemed to be grieving for lost hopes and objects.

Her relationship with the interviewer was particularly interesting. She developed an idealizing maternal transference which strongly suggested a curative fantasy in which she found the good mother whom she had so long sought.[15] The patient was astonished to discover that she could talk so openly to the interviewer and emphasized that she could never talk intimately to her own mother. She revealed secrets which she had told no one before. Evidence that she had internalized the therapist as a good object was revealed during the third session when she described an imaginary conversation at home with the interviewer during which she cried. Particularly striking to the patient was the fact that she was speaking in English, for she always thinks in her native language.

In her last session, the patient spoke very poignantly and with some desperation about the feeling of "deadness" which had overcome her in the last few years. She sought understanding and felt frustrated when it was not provided. A psychiatric referral was refused though the patient intimated that she would have liked to continue with the interviewer.

Comment

Though this woman lived a rich and vigorous life before she became ill, there was evidence of considerable conflict. She had intense oedipal attachments to both brother and father which resulted in sexual inhibition and probably participated in the failure of her only romantic love relationship. Most disturbing to her over the last few years is a feeling of "deadness." She describes this as a total absence of sexual desire or wish to be fondled or touched. The patient's uremic delusion that her fecal column was from a man reflects her derogation of women and identification with her brother and father. These masculine representations are important components of her ego ideal, and it is not surprising, therefore, to discover that there is a reversal of roles in her relationship with her husband.

It is of particular interest to trace the evolution of one of the dominant themes in her life, survivor guilt. Mrs. F was first troubled during the war by her need to conceal her identity and was well aware of the fact that many of the members of her family were killed. Her brother's death left her with the feeling that she was a survivor, particularly accentuated by the later awareness that she had received successful treatment for the same disease. The transplantation in particular evoked this theme. She wondered whether she should be alive after the transplant and was guilty that "the person who made her so happy was now dead" (a suggestive reference to the brother). Furthermore, the patient reexperienced guilt in the context of the rejection of the "twin kidney" in another patient; at which time, she made a potentially self-destructive error. The patient's current feeling of "deadness" may also relate to this guilt, although why it should have evolved in the past few years is not clear.

Although a depressive cloud colors her experience of life, she maintains her active stance and continues to struggle. The only ray of hope directed toward the future is connected with the fantasy of returning to Romania to visit her old lover.

This woman is the most difficult of all to evaluate. Though she is often unhappy, depressed, and dissatisfied with her current life, she maintains courage and a will to live. Previous renal disease and transplantation play a minimal role in her current preoccupations. She experiences moderate incapacitation from cardiac disease but actively seeks treatment.

It is impossible to predict what her life would have been like had she not become ill shortly after arrival in this country. How much is survivor guilt contributing to her failure to achieve satisfaction and contentment? Her story suggests that, apart from physical illness, she is confronted with an involutional crisis and despair related to her failure to fulfill earlier romantic aspirations and to achieve professional success which other life circumstances prevented her from achieving. Though clearly she has been affected by her physical illness, one must wonder whether her struggle would have been different had she not been ill. This woman poses all of the problems of outcome research which attempts to show relationships between earlier events and ultimate adaptation. The complexity of this woman's life experience defies easy dissection.

DISCUSSION

The extended interviews which we conducted with these patients offered a rich source of data about their life experiences in illness and health. Though no general conclusions can be drawn about long-term adaptation to illness, some comments can be made about the results and the problems inherent in this type of research.

The four-session evaluation with multiple interviews extended over time was of particular value in offering the patient an opportunity to elaborate his own preoccupations in life and his own thoughts about the illness and treatment experience. All of the patients required one or two sessions before they were free to respond spontaneously. A more structured interview situation might well have permitted greater reliability in focusing on very specific questions, but it would not have permitted the patient to convey the essence of his current life experience.

In general, a modification of Hamburg's criteria for adaptation to chronic illness,[16] was utilized to evaluate the quality of the patient's life. The following items were used as guidelines: (1) keeping distress within manageable limits and maintaining adequate sources of pleasure, (2) maintaining self-esteem, (3) maintaining adequate object relations, (4) working out to satisfaction personally valued and socially accepted roles, (5) maintaining some degree of hope for the future, (6) effecting rehabilitation to the patient's maximal physical capacity, and (7) maintaining an effective and reasonably trusting relationship with the treating physician. Utilizing these criteria, we came to convincing conclusions about the patient's current adaptation.

In each situation we formulated a trajectory of the patient's life situation and made estimates of the impact of the critical life events of illness, hemodialysis, and transplantation based upon the construction of a coherent life narrative. The present life structure of two of our patients (Mr. G and Mrs. D) appeared to be the natural continuation of their lives before illness began. Mr. G had matured considerably, was freer in the realm of physical activity, was progressing quite satisfactorily in the work he had begun before he became ill and was struggling to overcome dependency conflicts. The static quality of Mrs. D's life was characteristic of her personality, but she seemed quite happy as a married, though childless, suburban housewife. Though her complaint that she could not move to another part of the country was clearly an inhibition which she attributed to her illness, it was apparent that she was highly invested in remaining close to her parents. Both of these patients conveyed the sense that they were satisfied with the quality of their lives. In contrast, Mr. I was markedly maladapted and revealed depression and pervasive unhappiness. This represented a dramatic shift in his life trajectory and will be discussed below. Mrs. F was the most problematic of all the patients. Any adaptive rating scale would score her high on depression and unhappiness. Yet, this had a highly fluctuating character, and she retained a remarkable capacity to mobilize herself in order to overcome depression. Moreover, the unhappiness she described was related to the crisis of middle age and not to illness per se. Yet, in examining her life history, in recognizing that her illness began shortly after her migration to this country with its own privations and demands for adaptation, one cannot but wonder how much the experience of illness prevented her from utilizing her impressive strengths to rebuild a more satisfying life in her own country.

Although the original intent of the project was to evaluate the impact of transplantation on patients who retain their kidneys for over five years, it became apparent that this was not a question which could be answered directly. More pertinent is the question of what role transplantation plays in the lives of these patients at the present time. Clearly, we cannot assume that past recollections adequately reflect the actual experiences which the patients had undergone and the attitudes which they displayed at the time of transplantation.

What could be evaluated was the extent to which their lives were currently dominated by illness, by memories of illness, or by expectation of future illness. In essence, the focus shifted to become a study of the patients' lives, rather than of their illnesses, and it was not surprising to discover that other factors contributed strongly to whether they were happy or unhappy. The important issues varied considerably from patient to patient and related in part to the stages of the life cycle in which the patient found himself at the time of the transplant and at the present time. The small size of the sample limits meaningful generalizations and focuses attention on individual responses to stress and methods of coping. It became apparent that it was often difficult to obtain precise data about the patient's current perception of the kidney and fantasies about the kidney, particularly if the kidney appears to be well integrated in the body image. This was illustrated in the situation of Mr. I, who thought little about the kidney and had little anxiety about its loss until a recent hospitalization for cellulitis where a question was raised about diminishing the immunosuppressive medication in order to promote tissue healing. At this time, the threat of loss reactivated the representation of the kidney as a personified foreign body toward which he had a guilty obligation (a response characteristic of him when he received gifts).

Three of the four patients appeared to have integrated the transplanted kidney quite effectively into their body schema and experienced minimal current concern about loss. (It is our expectation that projective data will offer more information about this phenomenon.) One patient, Mrs. D, seven years after transplantation, revealed what Muslin[3] has called incomplete psychological internalization of the kidney which continued to be represented intrapsychically as a hostile introject.[11,14] Although the anxiety about loss which this generates is not severe, it does create a generally phobic attitude toward contact with physicians and the hospital, which potentially could lead to delay in her seeking medical attention. It has been pointed out that in addition to the intrapsychic effect of transplantation on this patient, the demand for a transplant from her sister has led to dramatic changes in the structure of the family relationships.

In summary, one can say that on a basis of the data obtained from four patients, no significant and pervasive fear of loss of the transplanted kidney persists.

The most difficult question to answer and the one which required the highest degree of inference pertained to the evaluation of the role of life experience and character as it influenced the impact of illness and transplantation on the current quality of life. Novey addresses this issue when he discusses the historical reconstruction as an intrinsic part of psychotherapy and psychoanalysis.[17] "An attempt is made to see the patient and to have him see himself in some continuing context in which his present modes of experiencing and dealing with himself and others are a logical outgrowth of previous experiences." He emphasizes that the total mass of evidence leads us to draw a certain conclusion because it has its own inherent logic and consistency, although he recognizes that certainty about a historical reconstruction is never possible.

Such a logic is present in the story of Mr. I who successfully coped with his early deprivation through independence and by giving to others. The adaptation was fragmented by illness, and his bitter litany of complaints of poor care and indifference reflect the return of feelings about his early experience. Similarly, Mrs. F's sense of loss and emptiness result from a failure in her romantic life which is a product of early incestuous inhibitions. Though these statements are admittedly interpretations, it is only through interpretation that one can make sense of one's life and of the lives of others.

Retrospective studies are subject to the criticism that conclusions can always be rationally explained and seen as logical outcomes based upon a manipulation of earlier data. It is interesting in this light to isolate elements in the past history of these patients which might have suggested different outcomes. Both Mr. G and Mrs. D had overprotective mothers whose prohibitions were internalized and remained active to the present day. In each case, there had been a particular gain in illness, yet neither of these patients maintained the sick role in a significant way.

Each of the four patients might have had significant dynamic reasons for continuing anxiety about kidney loss. Mrs. F behaved self-destructively when survivor guilt was activated at the time her "surgical twin" rejected the kidney. Currently, she describes no concern about the kidney loss. Mr. I's inability to take is tied to his avoidance of the feeling of guilty obligation but this has not led to preoccupation about kidney loss.

One of the generally postulated conditions for illness onset, object loss, was an important aspect of Mr. G's early life when his mother died—and his posttransplant course when his wife, who was a dependency object, decided to leave him. The grief which followed this loss was not accompanied by anxiety about loss of the kidney. Successful mourning may have protected the patient from this response. Even Mrs. D's failure to completely internalize the organ did not lead to a disabling preoccupation with loss.

One of the most interesting aspects of this study has been the unexpected intensity of the reaction of the patients to the interview situation. This was facilitated by the arrangement of weekly interviews extending over a month's time. Each of the patients came with a hidden agenda and seemed to be seeking a neutral person whom they could use as a confidant. They all behaved with the interviewer in ways which were characteristic of them and which gave an interesting perspective on their character structure. Transference reactions were evident, and, in one situation (Mrs. F), a latent curative fantasy developed which reflected her wish to find the idealized good mother. There were islands of loneliness in each of the patients which reflected their inability to communicate certain long-standing concerns to significant others. This acted as a strong motivation for participating in the research. It is impossible to say whether these reactions would be evoked in patients who had not been subject to such trying life experiences. In this light, each of the patients experienced what would reasonably be described as insights during these sessions. These insights had an emotional quality and offered new perspectives on the patient's previous life experience.

All of the patients requested reassurance and there were explicit and implicit demands for interpretation of aspects of their behavior. A considerable degree of flexibility was required in responding to the patient's questions and demands. It is clear that systematic plans to effect closure (i.e., to effect the equivalent of termination in a psychotherapy) must be part of future research using this technique. This will take the form of a presentation to the patient of a brief and tactful narrative of their lives showing the logic of their reactions to illness, hemodialysis, and transplantation. The patient will be allowed enough time to respond to the formulation, to modify it, and discuss it with us.

CONCLUSION

Final conclusions about the long-term psychological responses to renal transplantation await the study of a larger population. Initial findings suggest that patients have remarkable resiliency and ability to adapt to very trying and extraordinary circumstances. The extended interview has been very useful in obtaining the data which we seek. In our future studies this will be complemented by adaptive scales and projective tests. In the face of the patients' insistent demands for reassurance, interpretation, and understanding of their experience, we have decided to formulate and to present to them a simplified and tactful version of our understanding of their life experience based upon the information which they have given us. Clearly, what we say will be guided by our knowledge of defense and character style. We hope that this will add a dimension to both the patients' understanding and our understanding of what has been an extraordinary life experience for them.

REFERENCES

1. SIMMONS, R., KLEIN, S., and SIMMONS, R. Gift of life: the social and psychological impact of organ transplantation. New York: John Wiley and Sons, 1977.
2. MUSLIN, H. The kidney transplant patient: follow-up study. Presentation at Discussion Group, American Psychoanalytic Association, December 15, 1977.
3. MUSLIN, H. The emotional process of the kidney transplant: the process of internalization. Journal of the Canadian Psychiatric Association, 1972, 17, 553–558.
4. MUSLIN, H. On acquiring a kidney. American Journal of Psychiatry, 1971, 127, 1185–1188.
5. BEARD, B. The quality of life before and after renal transplantation, Diseases of the Nervous System, 1971, 32, 24–31.
6. ABRAM, H. The psychiatrist and the treatment of chronic renal failure and the prolongation of life. American Journal of Psychiatry, 1972, 128, 1534–1539.
7. GEORGE, J. P. Life with a transplanted kidney. The Medical Journal of Australia, March 7, 1970, 10, 461.
8. EISENDRATH, R. M. The role of grief and fear in the death of kidney transplant patient. American Journal of Psychiatry, 1969, 126(3), 381–387.
9. KEMPH, J. P. Kidney transplants and shifts in family dynamics. American Journal of Psychiatry, 1967, 125(5), 39–44.
10. KEMPH, J. P. Psychotherapy with donors and recipients of kidney transplants. Seminars in Psychiatry, 1971, 3(1), 145.
11. CASTELNUOVO-TEDESCO, P. Organ transplant, body image, psychosis. The Psychoanalytic Quarterly, 1973, 42(3), 349–363.
12. CROMBEZ, J. C. and LEFEBVRE, P. The behavioral responses of renal transplant patients as seen through their fantasy life. Canadian Psychiatric Association Journal, 1972,17, Suppl. 2:SS 19–72.
13. BASCH, S. H. The intraphysic integration of a new organ. The Psychoanalytic Quarterly, 1973, 42, 364–384.
14. VIEDERMAN, M. The search for meaning in renal transplantation. Psychiatry, 1974, 37, 283–290.
15. ORNSTEIN, P. H., and ORNSTEIN, A. On the continuing evolution of psychoanalytic psychotherapy. In Annual of Psychoanalysis, Vol. 5. New York, International Universities Press, 1977, pp. 329–370.
16. HAMBURG, D., and ADAMS, J. A Perspective on Coping Behavior. Archives of General Psychiatry, 1967, 17, 277–284.
17. NOVEY, S. The second look—the reconstruction of personal history in psychiatry and psychoanalysis. Baltimore: Johns Hopkins University Press, 1968.

20
Transplantation
Psychological Implications of Changes in Body Image

PIETRO CASTELNUOVO-TEDESCO

Among the reasons why transplants are of interest to psychiatrists and, in fact, to anyone concerned with psychological issues is that they touch on the phenomena of acute and chronic stress and of alteration of the body image.

Prior to the era of transplantation, our knowledge of body image dealt mainly with the external appearance of the body and was derived primarily from changes in the surface anatomy of the body, such as occur with amputations, phocomelias, and burns.[1] With the advent of transplants, on the other hand, new knowledge has been obtained about how the image of the interior of the body is organized psychologically.[2,3]

The term "body image," coined by Schilder in the 1930s,[4] derives from the observation that human beings develop and maintain a concept of the configuration of their bodies. We now realize that the body image is a very important part of the self-representation and closely related to the sense of who and what we are. Freud had anticipated this when he said (in *The Ego and the Id*) that the ego is first and foremost a body ego, meaning that the mental representation of the body—its shape, appearance, and characteristic functioning—is the very foundation of the ego itself.[5] Given this, it becomes very interesting to consider how this concept, the body image, is influenced when the architecture and anatomical arrangements of the body are radically and suddenly changed. I wish to note the following.

First, the body image is a fluid structure which is capable of giving up old parts and also of accepting new ones.[3,4] Normally, however, these changes only occur slowly and gradually.

Second, it takes time to adapt to changes in the body's architecture,

---

PIETRO CASTELNUOVO-TEDESCO, M.D. • James G. Blakemore Professor of Psychiatry, Vanderbilt University School of Medicine, Nashville, Tennessee.

especially if they occur suddenly. Evidence of this is provided by the phantom limb phenomenon. We know that after amputation it takes at least two to three years, and often many more than that, for phantom sensations to disappear.[1]

Third, a great deal of anxiety typically is associated even with the gradual changes in body image that normally occur over time, e.g., with aging. We know, for example, that men worry about losing their hair, women about acquiring wrinkles, and that both men and women exercise and seek the help of plastic surgeons to keep the inevitable changes in appearance from occurring too quickly. We know also how much concern is generated over these commonplace phenomena. If this, then, is the reaction to expectable and gradual changes, we easily can understand the much greater impact created by changes that occur suddenly and unexpectedly because of surgery or trauma.

Fourth, it makes a great deal of difference psychologically whether a body part is added or removed.[2,3] Each circumstance has psychological consequences that are entirely different. For this reason, we can now distinguish between two basic types of surgical interventions, "life-saving" and "life-extending" operations.[2,3,6]

"Life-saving" operations are the traditional ones, like an amputation or a gastrectomy, that *remove* a diseased body part. Because a part is lost, they bring about a *restriction* of the body image. The problems of adaptation to this kind of surgery typically are those of loss and depression and these reactions, to a mild degree at least, are quite routine after surgical intervention. Another characteristic of this form of surgery is that it permits the individual to reach, or at least approximate, his normal or "allotted" life span. All of us harbor the notion that we have been granted a certain life span, although we may be unwilling—consciously, perhaps—to state the years specifically. Typically, if we become ill, we are afraid that our life span may be shortened (we say, for example, that someone died "prematurely") and, by the same token, if we are successfully treated and recover, we assume that we will be able once more to reach our "allotted" life span (whatever it may be in the individual case). This view contrasts with the notion that the life span can be extended, which one finds in the setting of transplant surgery and which will be discussed shortly.

"Life-extending" operations are exemplified by transplant surgery. Here, typically, a body part from another human being is *added.* The body image is thus *enlarged* and a place has to be found for the new part which the body now comes to contain. Fundamentally, the transplanted organ is a foreign body which must be integrated into the body schema. Associated with this is the illusion that life has been extended beyond the "allotted" life span (since the patient would have died if he had not received the new part). In keeping with this illusion that life has been extended is the so-called rebirth phenomenon,[6,7] also referred to as the "second-chance phenomenon,"[8] which often is associated with a definite euphoria.[2,9] One notes, in contrast, that rebirth phenomena and euphoric reactions occur only very rarely after traditional surgery.

Now, the central point of this chapter. What happens psychologically when a new part is introduced into the body? How does this affect the body image?

First, the acquisition of a new organ is not just a matter of physiology—of the body adapting to the new part in purely physiological terms. The new organ is *not* psychologically inert. Rather it has psychological meaning and activity which it displays from the very beginning.[2,3,6] The realization that the organ comes from another person always has very serious implications. It leads typically to thoughts of having robbed the donor of a vital part so that the latter has been killed or injured. The form which these thoughts take obviously depends on the psychological integrity of the person, and will be presented most outspokenly when the recipient is in a highly regressed mental state. Certainly, with regression one readily finds evidence of primitive guilt and fears of punishment and retaliation.

For this reason, many patients prefer to receive a cadaver kidney rather than one from a related donor. A cadaver kidney helps to sidestep—but does not eliminate—the very difficult issue of indebtedness. A patient of mine, for example, said that he would rather receive a kidney from a cadaver than from his brother because—he added jokingly—if he and his brother ever had an argument, his brother might decide that he wanted his kidney back. This was a risk that the patient would rather not take.[2] Similarly, a patient with a heart transplant, whom I saw some years ago, postoperatively had an acute hallucinatory psychosis in which he thought that his donor, a woman, was coming back to retrieve her heart. In the midst of his psychosis the patient was not sure whether it was his heart or hers. Manifestations of merging and fusion were prominent.[6] In the same vein, Ferris[10] and Abram[7] have some evidence suggesting that patients who receive transplants from related donors are more likely to show psychologic complications than those who receive cadaver transplants.

In short, one finds that the transplant is not just a body part, but that psychologically it represents the whole person.[2,3,6,11,12,13] The recipient behaves as if now he had inside the donor himself. The process is somewhat as follows. After transplantation, the transplanted organ promptly achieves mental representation, i.e., it registers in the mind both as an anatomic part and as a symbolic representative of the donor. It also relates itself to existing introjects, especially those of the early parental figures. It unites with these and activates them. This renders the psychological situation of the patient potentially unstable, as shown by the relatively high incidence of emotional disturbance, depression, and occasionally psychosis after transplantation. Even if postoperatively the patient remains fully integrated psychologically, he often harbors the thought that he has acquired some crucial characteristic of the donor along with the kidney. This is evidence of the very powerful impact of the transplant experience. Identification with the donor is often, in fact, quite prominent. Patients often believe they have become more masculine or more feminine, depending on the sex of the donor.[8,11,13] This change is more or less acceptable, depending on whether recipient and donor are or are not of the same sex. It has been observed repeatedly that receiving an organ from a donor of the opposite sex can be quite upsetting for the recipient, especially if there are prominently unresolved issues of sexual identity. Patients have reported a variety of other traits which they believe (or are afraid) they have acquired from the donor as an outcome of transplantation. These include: generosity or altruism, artistic talent, religiosity, helpfulness, aggressiveness, capacity to speak a foreign language, physical size (e.g., slimness).[2,3,6,8,9,11-14] In other words, a host of characteristics or traits, both physical and psychological, have been thought by recipients to have been transmitted to them by the donors as a result of transplantation.

The traits of the donor with which the recipient identifies may be fantasied rather than real, and the phenomenon which just has been described is seen also in cases where the recipient receives a cadaver organ.[2,11,12] For example, a patient of mine who had received a cadaver kidney knew only about his donor that he had been a 38-year-old man. The patient assumed that the donor, because of his age, must have been married, with a family, and therefore stable and mature. From this the patient finally concluded that he had received from the donor a good measure of wisdom and common sense. The patient had a number of other thoughts concerning his donor which will not be reviewed here but are described in the original publication.[2] These clearly show how lively and intricate are the fantasies of recipients even about cadaver donors.

Because, as we have seen, the transplant is not a psychologically indifferent part, the issue of psychological compatibility with the donor becomes extremely important. Patients seek donors with whom they are psychologically compatible.[11,12] Thus, a patient of mine said that he would not want his brother's kidney because the brother was something of a "hippie" whereas the patient regarded himself as a "square." He felt sure, on this basis, that he would reject the brother's kidney.[2] Clinical examples highlighting this issue have been reported by various investigators. Basch, for example, mentions the case of a boy who made a suicidal gesture, went into rejection, and then died, after being told that his kidney came from his ne'er-do-well father, with whom he had always been at odds.[12] He simply wanted no part of his hated father and in his attempt to destroy the hated part, he destroyed himself. In other words, the quality of the relationship of recipient to donor seems to influence the outcome of the transplant and may contribute to possible rejection. The evidence on this point is not final but certainly is suggestive.[11,12,15]

The transplant, then, is not just a "piece of plumbing" but a symbolic representative of another human being and of the relationship, both real and fantasied, to that person. It is an anatomic part that has been anthropomorphized. After transplantation, the patient finds it difficult to regard the transplanted organ immediately as part of his body. Typically, he may report that it "feels funny," that it seems to "stick out." He is likely to regard it as fragile and needing special care; at first he is very protective of the new part and avoids any movement that conceivably might injure it.[13]

The integration of the transplanted organ into the patient's body schema requires time. Full integration of the new part is achieved only by some patients. Some accomplish it only partially and others not at all.[13,16] Finally, regardless of what degree of integration has been achieved, this can become reversed through regression at any time. One sees then a pathologic fusion of the ego boundaries of donor and recipient.[2,6,11,12] The evidence presented in this volume by Teschan, that even patients with functioning kidney transplants are likely to show EEG abnormalities, is most interesting. In this context, it provides a physiologic basis for the proneness that these patients have for psychological regression.

At some level, the patient views the transplant as something that does not belong to him and to which he has no rightful claim.[2,6,11,12] During regressed mental states, guilt about having "stolen" the organ may occur together with the feeling that his own essential characteristics have been altered as a result of possessing inside a part from another human being. Thus, early on some patients are euphoric and feel they have gained special strength as a result of this acquisition. Others, in a more regressed mental state, feel persecuted by the transplanted organ which they now regard as a malignant foreign body. Even during psychologically quiescent periods, there is a sense that, because of this potentially malignant foreign part, the patient is in a very vulnerable and unstable situation. Anxiety tends to be high and there is usually also a visible measure of depression. Typically, denial is massive and it is difficult for the patient to consider the broader aspects of his life situation. He has trouble giving thought to his prognosis and especially to making plans for the future. His outlook and his functioning are very much restricted to the here-and-now. Therefore, the psychotherapeutic help that the patient best can use is supportive in kind, whereas insight-oriented approaches often are poorly tolerated and prove rather unproductive.[18,19]

In conclusion, the emotional problems of transplantation are not simply a consequence of the ever-present possibility of malfunction or rejection. The issue of changed body image also creates much anxiety and makes transplantation a stressful and difficult solution to end-stage renal disease. These considerations bear on the continuing debate about the relative merits of dialysis and transplantation as long-term therapies for kidney failure. We should realize that transplantation contains a distinct potential for psychological complications which derives from the human source of the transplanted part and not just from the effectiveness with which the part functions. These formulations about body image again point to the patient's need for consistently supportive interactions and for a comprehensive approach to his problems—as we have been reminded by Dr. Chad Calland,[20] the physician with renal disease who wrote so thoughtfully about the plight of the renal patient.

REFERENCES

1. KOLB, L. D. Disturbances of the body image. In S. Arieti (Ed.), *American handbook of psychiatry*. Vol. 1. New York: Basic Books, 1975.
2. CASTELNUOVO-TEDESCO, P. Organ transplant, body image, psychosis. *Psychoanalytic Quarterly*, 1973, 42, 349–363.
3. CASTELNUOVO-TEDESCO, P. Ego vicissitudes in response to replacement or loss of body parts. Certain analogies to events during psychoanalytic treatment. *Psychoanalytic Quarterly*, 1978, 47, 381–397.
4. SCHILDER, P. *The image and appearance of the human body*. New York: International Universities Press, 1950.
5. FREUD, S. (1923) *The ego and the id*. *Standard edition*, Vol. 19, London: Hogarth Press, 1961, pp. 3–66.
6. CASTELNUOVO-TEDESCO, P. Psychoanalytic considerations in a case of cardiac transplantation. In S. Arieti (Ed.), *The world biennial of psychiatry and psychotherapy*. Vol. 1. New York: Basic Books, 1971, pp. 336–352.
7. ABRAM, H. S., and BUCHANAN, D. C. The gift of life: a review of the psychological aspects of kidney transplantation. *International Journal of Psychiatry in Medicine*, 1976–77, 7, 153–164.
8. CRAMOND, W. A. Renal homotransplantation—some observations on recipients and donors. *British Journal of Psychiatry*, 1967, 113, 1223–1230.
9. KEMPH, J. P. Psychotherapy with patients with kidney transplant. *American Journal of Psychiatry*, 1967, 124, 623–629.
10. FERRIS, G. N. Psychiatric considerations in patients receiving cadaveric renal transplants. *Southern Medical Journal*, 1969, 62, 1482–1484.
11. VIEDERMAN, M. The search for meaning in renal transplantation. *Psychiatry*, 1974, 37, 283–290.
12. BASCH, S. H. The intrapsychic integration of a new organ: a clinical study of kidney transplantation. *Psychoanalytic Quarterly*, 1973, 42, 364–384.

13. MUSLIN, H. On acquiring a kidney. *American Journal of Psychiatry*, 1971, *127*, 1185–1188.
14. TIME MAGAZINE. A new kidney from Moscow. 1977, *March 7*, p. 84.
15. VIEDERMAN, M. Psychogenic factors in kidney transplant rejection: A case study. *American Journal of Psychiatry*, 1975, *132*, 957–959.
16. BIORK, G., and MAGNUSSON, G. The concept of self as experienced by patients with a transplanted kidney. *Acta Medica Scandinavica*, 1968, *183*, 191–192.
17. TESCHAN, P. E. This volume.
18. BUCHANAN, D. This volume.
19. FREYBERGER, H. This volume.
20. CALLAND, C. Iatrogenic problems in end-stage renal failure. *New England Journal of Medicine*, 1972, *287*, 334–336.

21

Psychological Reactions to Giving a Kidney

ROBERTA G. SIMMONS

INTRODUCTION

Kidney transplantation involves the unique resource of donated kidneys. Both living relatives and "newly dead cadavers" can provide this resource, with a living relative donating one of his kidneys to save the life of a family member and with cadavers able to donate both kidneys to persons on a waiting list. Because of immunological processes, the living related kidneys have tended to do better and survive longer;[1] in addition, patients with willing related donors are spared the long and uncertain time on a waiting list. However, there is a widespread skepticism about the ability of a relative to make the major sacrifice of a kidney willingly and without significant regret later on.[2] The perception is that family blackmail and pressure will be pervasive and will be the major factor motivating the potential donor. Posttransplant, the loss of a body part will engender long-term regret and depression. Thus, at many centers the policy of using related donors is regarded as a major ethical problem.[3,4]*

Over the past few years we have attempted to evaluate the psychological effects of donation upon related donors to see (1) how frequent and how willing volunteering is, and (2) to explore the psychological consequences of giving up a body part. What are the costs and gains of related donation? How do these costs and gains compare to those of the alternatives?[7-9]

---

*Physicians are also wary of subjecting a normal person to even the small risk of donation. For information concerning risk and complications, see references 5 and 6.

ROBERTA G. SIMMONS, PH.D. • Professor of Sociology and Psychiatry, University of Minnesota, Minneapolis, Minnesota.

METHOD

To explore the impact of donation on the related donor and his family, we collected the following data at the University of Minnesota: (1) Between 1970 and 1973 we administered questionnaires to all 130 related donors pretransplant, and again at five days posttransplant, and at one year posttransplant if the kidney was still functioning; (2) between 1970 and 1973 the entire cohort of 178 adult transplant recipients were interviewed at three comparable times; (3) between 1970 and 1972 we followed the entire cohort of 205 families intensively over time; and (4) between 1970 and 1972 we administered questionnaires to 186 family members who could have volunteered but did not do so ("nondonors"). These "nondonors" were interviewed at a month posttransplant when the transplanted kidney was still functioning.[7]

In addition, in a more recent follow-up in 1978–79 we have interviewed all living related donors in the above cohort whether or not the transplant was still successful. These last interviews bring the cohort to five to nine years posttransplant.

Finally, in an exploratory study, 14 families who donated kidneys from "cadaver donors" were interviewed intensively at least a year after the donation.[7]

Thus, these studies collected both quantitative and in-depth qualitative information. In terms of the quantitative information, self-esteem and depression–happiness items and scales were derived from well-known sources;[10] the scales were constructed from many multiple choice items. For the scales, reliability was satisfactory as measured by Cronbach's alpha and the self-esteem scale has been extensively validated.[7]

For the in-depth material, two independent raters categorized much of the material pertaining to the donor search and the family. Where used, the reliability was satisfactory.

RESULTS

Pretransplant

Our findings point to a much greater willingness to donate an organ than is assumed by the lay or medical public. Family members are surprisingly willing to make this major sacrifice to save the life of a loved one. Out of all eligible family members, 57% volunteered to donate and took the definite preliminary step of having their blood tested (see Table 1). Furthermore, the vast majority of those who did donate reported little or

TABLE 1
Volunteering to Donate by Family Relationship of Eligible Donor

	Mother	Father	Daughter	Son	Sister	Brother	Total
Donated or volunteered	86%	86%	66%	66%	48%	46%	57%
Did not volunteer	14%	14%	33%	34%	52%	54%	43%
Total	100%	100%	100%	100%	100%	100%	100%
	(74)	(70)	(54)	(66)	(217)	(237)	(815)

no ambivalence related to the basic decision to donate, although concerns about the surgery were not infrequent.

In the majority of cases the decision to donate was an immediate, instantaneous one, made with no deliberation and usually with no later regret. In order to arrive at this conclusion, two independent coders coded the decision process taking into account both the story of the donor and that told by other relatives.[7,11] The following quotations capture the process of instantaneous decision-making:

Case 1
> DONOR (MOTHER): Me? I never thought about it. . . . I automatically thought I'd be the one. There was no decision to make or sides to weigh.

Case 2
> DONOR'S WIFE: You mean did he think about it and then decide? No—it was just spontaneous. The minute he knew . . . it was just natural. The first thing he thought of. He would donate.

Case 3
Interview with donor (sister)
> INTERVIEWER: Who told you about the need for a donor?
> DONOR: [The recipient.] I came back from my vacation. She picked me up at the plane. I knew something was bothering her. After Dad went to bed I said "OK, what's bugging you?" The evening was fraught with emotion.
> INTERVIEWER: What was your initial reaction?
> DONOR: The initial reaction was, "Of course, I'll do it."
> INTERVIEWER: [later] When did you make your final decision to donate a kidney?
> DONOR: I don't think it was a decision. I really didn't consider much. I kept thinking "What was the decision?" My sister kept saying I had to make a decision. I kept thinking what was I supposed to be thinking about? As far as I was concerned . . . I would donate a kidney.

Interview with recipient about the first time she mentioned a transplant to her sister
> INTERVIEWER: Do you remember what you said to her at the time?
> RECIPIENT: I think I told her that I had a choice of going on the machine or having a transplant. I didn't have to say much because she

[knows something about medicine] and . . . is just one of these gals, and said immediately that she would do it.

Case 4
Interview with recipient
INTERVIEWER: Who first talked to the donor about the transplant?
RECIPIENT: My husband and I. She visited often. She came in when I was still crying right after the doctor told me. She said, "Don't worry. You can have mine." I thought after she thought about it she might change her mind, but she didn't.
INTERVIEWER: How long did it take for the donor to decide to donate?
RECIPIENT: A couple of seconds when she found out about it.
When the donor in this case was asked the same question, she said:
DONOR: I didn't think about it. That's what I'm here for.

The instantaneous character of the decision to donate a kidney has also been reported by Fellner and Marshall in their smaller series.[12,13]

Was there untoward family pressure to donate in our series? According to two independent coders, unwelcome direct family pressure occurred for only 11% of the donors. However, more subtle pressures appear inevitable. The donor frequently learned of the need for donation in the presence of his dying relative, and volunteering at such an instant would probably appear highly desirable, especially to a relative who was already positively oriented. Feelings of family obligation were common but appeared to make the decision easier rather than more difficult. The obligation to sacrifice for one's family was widely accepted as legitimate among those donors, and those who felt more obligated were also likely to be the more willing donors.[7]

DONOR (BROTHER): I guess I see it as my Christian duty . . . and brotherly love.

DONOR (GRANDMOTHER): It kind of scares you but . . . we try to do whatever we can for her; after all, I'm her grandmother.

Posttransplant

Posttransplant, the vast majority of donors indicated they were without regret, and in fact were extremely happy that they had donated and that the recipient was alive and healthier. They felt closer to the patient, an emotion that was warmly reciprocated (Table 2). Most donors received a great deal of family praise and gratitude both before and after.

Most interesting is the finding that donors' global self-esteem and level of depression–happiness improved after the transplant, and that these improved feelings of happiness persisted to a year posttransplant (Table 3). Although the level of happiness of the donor pretransplant was similar to that of normal control groups, the level at a year posttransplant

TABLE 2
Closeness between Recipient and Donor

| | Percent reporting they feel "very close"[a] to the other | |
	According to donor	According to recipient
Pretransplant	59%	55%
Shortly after transplant[b]	77%	86%
One year posttransplant[b]	71%	77%

[a]The multiple choice question was, "Would you say that you are very close, somewhat close, a little close, or not at all close to _____?"
[b]These questions were asked for cases in which the donated kidney was still functioning.

TABLE 3
Comparison of Individual Donor's Scores on Self-Esteem[a] and
Depression–Happiness over Time

Comparison of	Donor's score becomes worse over time	Donor's score stays the same	Donor's score improves over time	Total
Self-esteem pretransplant and 5 days posttransplant	27%	27%	45%	100% (113)
Self-esteem pretransplant and 1 year posttransplant	33%	29%	38%	100% (97)
Depression–happiness pretransplant and 5 days posttransplant	17%	35%	48%	100% (109)
Depression–happiness pretransplant and 1 year posttransplant	24%	32%	44%	100% (93)

[a]Corrected nine-item donor self-esteem scale.

exceeded that of these groups (Table 4). In Table 4 we see that pretransplant 34% of the donors and 30–37% of the control groups scored high in happiness. However, a year after the transplant 60% of the donors scored high in happiness according to this measure.

These matters were collected following an interview about the donation and the transplant, and these improvements in the self-image and happiness–depression might have been less evident if the questionnaire were administered in a situation unrelated to the donation. Nevertheless, when the transplant is made salient, there is evidence that the donors think more highly of themselves and are happier than they were pretransplant. In-depth interviews also demonstrate a great exhilaration on the part of many donors when they speak of the gift a year later:

TABLE 4
Happiness of Donors and Control Groups

	Donor			Controls, Twin City[a]		National control[b]		
		One year						
	Pretransplant	posttransplant	Nondonors	Control 1	Control 2	1963	1963	1965
Taken all together how would you say things are these days? Would you say you are:								
Very happy[c]	34%	60%	26%	37%	37%	36%	32%	30%
Pretty happy	58%	35%	68%	54%	56%	55%	51%	53%
Not too happy	8%	5%	5%	9%	6%	9%	16%	17%
Total	100%	100%	100%	100%	100%	100%	100%	100%
	(134)	(111)	(174)	(75)	(75)	(2460)	(1501)	(1460)

[a] The entire study in which these samples were used is reported in Simmons et al.[22]
[b] Bradburn, 1969, p. 40.[23]
[c] According to a chi-square analysis of the difference among the two donor groups and nondonors, p <.001.

INTERVIEWER: Why would you encourage someone to donate?
DONOR: (donated to sister) To save a person's life makes you feel like a better person. There are rewards.

DONOR: (donated to sister) I think I see myself as a little more human and patient. Just the fact of giving part of my body . . . and donating to someone who's going to live because of it . . . I guess I consider it one of the more worthwhile experiences of my life.

INTERVIEWER: How do you generally feel now about having donated?
DONOR: (donated to mother) Great! It's fantastic to see. When I lived with her she was [always] sick. It's great to see how healthy she is now and to see her happy! And grateful!

INTERVIEWER: What words would you use to describe a living relative who donates a kidney?
DONOR: (donated to sister) It's a wonderful feeling, that's all.

Thus, far from pointing to a major psychological cost of donation, these results suggest that donation may in fact have sizeable social–emotional benefits. Many donors think more highly of themselves after having saved the life of a relative.

Despite this benign picture for the majority of donors, at all points in time there appeared to be a small group of donors who were extremely ambivalent or regretful of their decision (5–8% depending on the measure used),[7] e.g.,

DONOR (BROTHER): (donated to sister) Like it's caused me to worry. This dumb thing has turned me into a hypochondriac. Now everytime I get sick I worry "Why am I getting sick? Maybe my kidney is flipping out."

If the donation was not successful and the transplant was rejected, the proportion expressing regret rose to 18%.[9,14] However, in both success and failure, the vast majority of donors do not express significant regret at donation. Even where the kidney failed the majority were glad they had attempted to save the patient:

BROTHER: (donated to adult brother who died one month later) Just to sum it all up, knowing what I do know now, I'd still do it even though I knew he wasn't going to make it. It was the right thing for him to know his brothers were backing him.

FATHER: (donated to daughter) Just the fact that you are able to help somebody . . . it's the feeling that . . . if anything . . . I feel at least I tried.

SON: (donated to mother) I was disappointed . . . I had great expectation of it working. Nobody had no control over what happened. It just happened . . . I'm glad that I tried because if I wouldn't have, and if I'd held back, I would've been haunted by the fact that she might've been saved.

Although in the vast majority of families, recipients and donors end up with intensified feelings of closeness, there is a small minority of cases where the donation caused significant difficulties between recipient and donor.[15] According to answers to multiple choice questions, 7% of recipients and 6% of donors indicate that their relationship has become difficult because of the transplant, and 20% of the recipients tell us they feel uncomfortable that they cannot pay the donor back. Although family difficulties due to the donation are not common, they tend to be dramatic when they occur:

> DONOR (SISTER): (donated to brother) I would say for three months [the recipient] tried to avoid me. I was never so crushed. I would call him up and he would be as cold as ice. I was destroyed. To this day I don't mention the kidney in front of him. Whenever I do, it turns him off. He has never come out and said "Thank you."

Which Donors Benefit Most? Which Benefit Least?

While no one factor was highly predictive, some donors reacted more favorably to the donation than others. In order to investigate the correlates of negative and positive feelings toward donation, several scales were created from multiple choice items: a scale of pretransplant ambivalence, of negative feelings and regret about donation at five days and at a year posttransplant,* and a scale measuring the extent to which the donor feels he is a better and more worthwhile person and more heroic because he has donated—the "better person" scale. The exact scales and their coefficients of reliability are presented in Simmons et al.[7]

Five major factors appear to be related to the donor's response to this experience: (1) his background and family statuses; (2) his interpersonal, emotional relationships within the family; (3) his personality pretransplant, (4) his pretransplant attitude toward donation, and (5) his concerns about the patient's prognosis. (See Table 5 for a summary of these factors.)

Family Statuses

Sex Roles. The male donor's reaction to donation is very different from the female donor's reaction. Prior to the transplant the male is more likely to be ambivalent than is the female ($r = .23$, $p = .007$). Posttransplant males persist in having more negative feelings toward dona-

---

*Although only a few donors have *extremely* negative feelings, donors do differ in the degree of postiveness or negativeness they feel, and these scales attempt to capture such differences.

TABLE 5
Donors Reacting Less Positively to Donation

Status
  Males
  Nonparents
  Among siblings and children, those who are married
Emotional relationship
  Persons less close to the patient
  "Black sheep" donors
  Persons who do not receive gratitude from family and patient
Personality
  Less-happy persons
  Persons with lower self-esteem
Less-obligated donors
  Not "only possible" donors
  Not A-match donors
Prior attitude
  Persons with high ambivalence to donation pretransplant

tion both at five days $(r = .22, p = .008)$ and a year after the event $(r = .20,$ $p = .02)$.

However, not all males react to donation negatively, and those who do not are more likely than are females to rate themselves as better persons after the transplant. At five days posttransplant 23% of males versus 8% of females score high in the "better person" scale $(p = .03)$, and this difference persists to a year posttransplant (40% vs. 26%).

What these results suggest is that donation is a more momentous event for the male. He is more likely to question whether he wishes to make this sacrifice. If he does make the sacrifice, he reacts more dramatically—either with regret or with a great boost in the self-picture. The female appears to take donation more for granted, neither reacting as negatively nor as likely to perceive the act to be an extraordinary one on her part, as an act that proves her to be a greater person.

Perhaps donation seems to the female to be a simple extension of her usual family obligations, while for the male it is an unusual type of gift. In our society the traditional female role is one in which altruism and sacrifice within the family is expected; the female is the customary family nurse and caretaker in times of illness and need.[16]

In fact, entering a hospital and suffering pain and body manipulation to give life to another is ordinarily a major part of her role and purpose in life. Giving birth to an infant is congruent psychologically with the act of giving a body part so a loved one can be reborn, so he can have a "second chance at life." The imagery of rebirth, of helping a person to be reborn, occurs frequently in conversations with transplant families, as Rapaport noted in *A Second Look at Life*.[17]

From a male's point of view, there is no life experience or expectation like childbirth that prepares him for this act of donation. Thus he may have stronger ambivalences and doubts even after the transplant. In any case, whether his feelings are positive or negative, he is more likely to feel he has performed an exceptional act. If his feelings are positive, as the majority of men's are, he is more likely to reap self-image benefits from this extraordinary gift.

Other Family Statuses. Donation is an extreme example of family help-giving behavior. The question arises as to the strength of the ties among blood relatives in the American family. In terms of cultural definition, the expectation that *parents* will aid and sacrifice for their children is indeed a strong one. The obligation of adult siblings to one another or of adult children to their parents would appear much less clear.

Parents are less ambivalent than other family donors ($r = -.21$, $p = .01$) and have less negative feelings about donation immediately after the transplant ($r = -.15, p = .06$), although this difference disappears a year later. Overall, brothers and sons are more negative than other relatives. In terms of a perceived boost in the self-picture, parents do not differ consistently from other donors in their scores on the "better person" scale.

In the case where siblings and children are used as donors, more than one family unit is likely to be involved. The donors, if married, are members both of their family of origin and their family of procreation. Some donors feel caught between obligations to these two families, between obligations to the recipient and to their own spouse and children who are dependent upon their continued health. The power of this conflict is reflected in a comparison of the feelings of married and unmarried donors. Siblings and children, if married, are more likely than their unmarried counterparts to be ambivalent donors ($r = .19, p = .06$), and to report negative feelings at a year posttransplant ($r = .35, p = .002$). Other data indicate that siblings and children who are married also perceive themselves to be less close to the recipient than do the unmarried donors.

One other characteristic of a person's status in the family involves the presence or absence of other potential donors. If an individual believes he is the only possible donor in the family, the obligation he feels to donate might be stronger. Does such a donor require additional protection from the medical staff to prevent him from donating under duress? Although such donors are slightly more likely to be ambivalent pretransplant ($r = .12$) and at five days posttransplant ($r = .10$), they are no more likely than others to demonstrate negative feelings at a year after the transplant. In fact, donors who are the only possible donors are more likely than others to believe that donation has improved their worthiness as individuals. They are more likely to score high on the "better person" scale at five days ($r = .27, p = .002$) and slightly more likely a year posttransplant ($r = .10$). Thus, these data would not support any *a priori* exclusion of such donors, although in any screening process they are slightly more likely to appear among those initially more ambivalent and requiring consideration.

Emotional Family Relationships

The most obvious hypothesis is that persons who feel closer to the patient pretransplant will be particularly desirous of donating and will maintain the most positive attitudes over the long run. In truth the data support this reasoning, although the correlations are not large. The correlation between closeness to the patient and ambivalence is $-.14$ ($p = .08$), between closeness and short-term negative feelings $-.18$ ($p = .02$) and for long-term negative attitudes $-.20$ ($p = .03$). Because parents and females are closer to the patient than others, the question arises whether closeness to the patient remains an important correlate of later adjustment if we control for these factors. Above and beyond parenthood and being a female relative, closeness still matters, but to a smaller extent. Donors who report they are closer to the patient are still less likely to show negative feelings at any time after the transplant ($r = .12$, $p = .09$ for five days; $r = .16$ for negative feelings at one year). Prior closeness to the patient appears to have no effect upon the donor's perception of himself as a more worthy person.

Moving from the donor's emotional relationship with the recipient to his interpersonal role within the entire family, we are led to examine the impact of the donation on the "black sheep" donor. There are few true "black sheep," but there are many donors whose past included a major act that met family disapproval. Here the broad conception of "black sheep" is used, and both those who presently are subject to family disapproval and those whose past led to problems are included. It is possible that such "black sheep" have donated in order to compensate for past wrongs; and the issue is what effect donation has upon them.

"Black sheep," though not clearly more ambivalent prior to the transplant, do end up with slightly more negative feelings posttransplant ($r = .13$, $p = .08$ at five days; and $r = .16$, $p = .07$ at a year).* Although right after the transplant, "black sheep" donors are slightly less likely than others to perceive themselves as better persons due to the donation ($r = -.11$),* this difference disappears by a year.

*This partial correlation between "black sheep" status and attitude toward donation holds constant whether or not the donor was the recipient's parent and regardless of the donor's sex. This control is necessary because males and nonparents are more likely to be "black sheep."

Thus in the long-run the "black sheep" donor is somewhat more likely than other relatives of his type and sex to react negatively. Perhaps the desire to compensate for past wrongs and to reinstate their position in the family is not likely to be as successful as hoped for by such donors.

The tendency to perceive oneself as a better person after donation appears to be a response to the amount of gratitude one's family expresses after the transplant. That is, those donors who report receiving more *explicit gratitude* from patient and family are more likely to indicate that donation has rendered them a better person. The correlations between the score on the "better person" scale and reported expression of gratitude from the family are .11 at five days and .30 ($p = .001$) a year later. At a year posttransplant the donor is also less likely to have negative feelings about donation if the family has explicitly thanked him since the transplant ($r = -.22, p = .01$), and if the recipient has done likewise ($r = -.18, p = .03$).

Personality

The donor's self-esteem and general level of depression–happiness was measured when he or she first entered the hospital for a work-up. These pretransplant measures do not correlate with ambivalence to donation before the transplant, but they are significantly associated with the donor's posttransplant reaction, although many of the correlations are not large. Patients who appear to be less *happy* or more depressed in general prior to the transplant have more negative feelings to donation a year later ($r = .27$, $p = .005$). Also, initially *low self-esteem* is associated with negative feelings immediately after the transplant ($r = .14, p = .07$), but this difference does not persist. Persons with low self-esteem prior to donation are slightly less likely to report that the donation has made them better persons at both points in time ($r = .10$ and .08).

Thus persons most in need of improvement in the self-picture are not the ones most likely to perceive the donation as having this particular effect. In fact, a negative attitude toward one's life during the pretransplant period appears to generalize to the specific posttransplant attitude toward donation. A generally negative self-attitude pretransplant places one at somewhat greater risk in terms of reaction to the donation event.

Prior Attitude to Donation

Another predictor of negative attitudes posttransplant is the donor's *specific attitude to donation* pretransplant. The correlations between pretransplant ambivalence and negative feelings at five days is .15 ($p = .06$),

and between ambivalence and negative feelings at a year is .31 (p = .001).*
Long-term improvements in the self-picture, as measured by the "better
person" scale, are not affected, however, by pretransplant ambivalence.
Ambivalent donors are not less likely than others to experience this
benefit of donation.

While ambivalence prior to the transplant may alert one to more
vulnerable donors, the lack of a *very* high correlation indicates that many
persons who are ambivalent pretransplant react positively after the operation is over.

Concerns about the Patient's Prognosis

One type of donor—the A-match family member—presents particular ethical problems. A transplant with an A-match kidney almost always
is successful, with better than 90% of patients showing long-term kidney
survival. If the patient surmounts early infection problems in the first year
and if there are no technical difficulties, the physicians expect almost
indefinite kidney function. Thus the A-match donor, who is almost
always a sibling, is likely to be under particular pressure to donate. Does
such a patient require special protection psychologically? Contrary to
expectation, A-match donors are *less* likely than others to indicate am-
bivalance (r = −.17, p = .07, controlling for type of relative). In addition,
after the transplantation the A-match donor reacts much like the individual who perceives himself to be the only possible donor. Both types of
donors may feel more obligated than others to donate, and the evidence
shows that both types react more positively posttransplant than do others
who were less obligated. At a year after the transplant, the A-match
donor is less likely than others to demonstrate negative feelings
(r = −.16, p = .05, controlling for type of relative).

The greater expectation of success on the part of the A-match donor
is probably largely responsible for their lower ambivalence and fewer
negative feelings. In worrying about the protection of donors who are
under special obligation to donate (the A-match donor and the only
possible donor) one ought not to discount the possibility that a strong
obligation may lessen the likelihood that the donor will have second
thoughts. The donor may more easily regard his sacrifice positively if he
believes his duty was strong. If other relatives would have been as
adequate a donor as he, the fact that he voluntarily placed himself in
jeopardy may cause some psychological discomfort.

For all donors, not only A-match donors, the patient's level of health
at a year after the transplant is important. We asked the donor at a year:

---

*If sex and type of relative are controlled, the correlations are reduced to .09 and .29
(p = .004).

240   ROBERTA G. SIMMONS

In recent months would you say the transplant patient has been (1) very
healthy, (2) somewhat healthy, (3) a little healthy, or (4) not at all healthy.

Donors who perceive the patient as more healthy tend to have slightly
less negative attitudes toward the transplant ($r = -.12$). The sacrifice has
not been in vain.

Before summarizing this section, we should examine the effect of one
additional factor upon the donor's response to donation—that is, his age.
Ethical questions have been raised about the use of minors as donors. Are
they truly capable of informed consent? The use of older donors, aged 50
and above, has also been questioned because they are likely to be greater
surgical risks. In our previous work[18,19] we have demonstrated that these
two groups are likely to have very positive attitudes toward donation,
both before and after the transplant. In the cohort described here, 23
donors aged 16–21 have been used, as have 25 donors aged 50 and above.
Although age differences do not show consistent patterns, the youngest
and oldest donors are surely no more likely than others to have negative
attitudes toward donation. In fact, if anything, the ones with the most
negative attitudes appear to be those in their late 20s and 30s, the life cycle
stages of childbearing and nurturing. The youngest and oldest donors are
usually free from obligation to care for young children. The donation and
the threat to their health does not place their own family at the same level
of risk.

The youngest donors complain much less of soreness right after the
transplant than does any other group, even those in their mid and late
twenties. In a review of 26 adolescents worked-up for donation, 18 of
whom were used, Bernstein and Simmons[18] also indicate that the majority of adolescents appeared to be under no blatant family pressure to
donate. Seventy-three percent of the potential donors in the series (21 out
of 26) and 89% of the actual donors (16 out of 18) were subject to no undue
pressure. In many cases, in fact, parents tended to protect the adolescent
from the surgical process and either hesitated to ask about donating or
were opposed to donation until convinced by the adolescent himself. Of
the five potential donors classified as experiencing some pressure, only
three experienced more than mild pressure. The first case involved a
retarded schizophrenic teenager who was excluded by the staff on
psychiatric grounds. The second was also not used as a donor but had
been pressured in favor of donation by one parent, while the other was
opposed to her donation. The third case was a "black sheep" donor who
felt rejected by the parents who wished him to donate.

Out of all the adolescent donors, only one indicated long-term emotional difficulty. This was a donor who pretransplant had agreed to talk to
the sociologists only after being assured that his ambivalence would not
be reported to the medical staff who might then prevent his donation to
his sister. Subsequent to the donation he indicated fear of developing

kidney disease and required short-term therapy for a depressive reaction about a month after the transplant. At a year this fear still remained, as did some turmoil with his family.

A more typical adolescent reaction at a year after the donation is the following:

> DONOR: The kids at school said I had guts [and] they don't. My parents said it was thoughtful and there was a lot of hugging that never happened before. They didn't think I could do it because of my age.

Summary

In this analysis the types of donors who are more likely to react negatively have been identified. Males appear more likely than females to treat the donation as a momentous occurrence; they show more extreme negative *and* positive reactions. Relatives other than parents, particularly brothers and sons, are more likely to respond negatively, especially if they are married and have obligations to a family of their own. Holding constant the nature of the blood relationship to the patient (that is, whether or not the donor is the recipient's parent), the following types of donors are less likely to respond positively: donors who pretransplant are emotionally less close to the patient, "black sheep" donors, individuals who do not receive explicit gratitude from the family after the transplant, persons who show low happiness and low self-esteem on pretransplant personality measures, and donors who demonstrate marked ambivalence before the operation. Donors who believe the patient is not doing well at a year also have more negative feelings about the donation. In addition, certain other donors are more likely to react well to the experience: relatives who are more obligated to donate because they are an A-match or the only possible donor. Neither the donors' education nor income predict their adjustment to donation.

Finally, we should note that even the donors who appear to be most vulnerable frequently react postively to the experience, and some donors have negative reactions that could not be foreseen. The fact that extremely negative reactions are rare while positive ones are frequent must be taken into account in any attempt to exclude donors on psychological grounds.

Cadaver Donor Families

The major alternative to donation from relatives is donation from cadavers. What is the psychological reaction of families who have donated organs from a member who has died suddenly and unexpectedly?

TABLE 6
Ratings of Attitudes of Cadaver-Donor Family Members
One Year or More after the Donation[a]

Attitude	Adults		Children under 14	Total	
Clearly positive	(17)	60% ⎫	(7)	(24)	68% ⎫
		⎬ 82%			⎬ 85%
Primarily positive with	(6)[b]	22% ⎭		(6)	17% ⎭
a few slight reservations					
Ambivalent	(1)	4%		(1)	3%
Negative	(4)[c]	14%		(4)	11%
Total	(28)	100%	(7)	(35)	100%

[a] Two of the authors made these ratings independently.
[b] Four out of six of these persons are from the same family.
[c] Two of these persons are from the same family.

Due to our small sample of 14 families, these findings must be regarded as more tentative than those concerning related donors.[20]

Table 6 shows that the reaction of members of cadaver donor families is much like that of related donors. The vast majority show positive attitudes, but a small minority (11–14%) report negative feelings and regret.

In making the decision to donate and in their later reactions, family members report both positive and negative factors. Frequent factors motivating the key family members toward donation were their empathy with the ill kidney recipients, their desire for some type of physical immortality for their own relative, and their desire that the death of their young relative have some meaning. At the same time, the decision and the period following the decision were sometimes made more stressful because the relatives had difficulty in accepting the concept of brain death when the cadaver appeared to be breathing and when his heart was still beating. They experienced uncertainty when no exact moment of death could be identified in other than an arbitrary way. Despite the fact they had been told the patient was dead, some relatives felt guilty at having to sign the papers that guaranteed his removal from the machinery maintaining his heartbeat.

The following quotations capture both those positive and negative attitudes.

Positive Feelings

The death was not a total loss. There was something good that came out of the whole thing.

I feel good about the transplant. I'm sure we did the right thing.

We decided to donate so he could keep living somehow.

If we can't save him, we can save someone else.

I feel good knowing that somebody got some benefit from his death, that there not only was a divine reason for it, but that there was something else, something tangible, that somebody profited some way.

I feel like part of him lives in somebody else. I really feel that he has done well for himself, that he gave all that he could give in his life and his death.

Maybe that's why he was here, or something. Maybe the other children [recipients] will do something, make a contribution or something.

Negative Feelings

The following mothers of cadaver donors noted the difficulty of accepting brain death. In both cases, the individual was dead, but machinery kept the heart beating and the cadaver apparently breathing. Only when the parent signed permission for donation would the kidneys be removed and then the machinery discontinued.

For the most part, people said, "Well, great." They thought it [the donation] was a tremendous thing to do. But I think the majority of them say this not knowing that you give up their organs before their heart has stopped beating. My mother died seven months before he [son] did and I stood at her bedside and felt her pulse until it was completely gone. It's a different kind of thing when you walk into a room and see the kid is breathing. You know the difference.

There he was right around the corner, still breathing on a machine and we were signing his life away in here.

CONCLUSION

Thus, our studies indicate positive psychological reactions on the part of the majority of related donors as well as gains in the recipient–donor relationship. Against these positive reactions of the majority and against the physical benefit to the recipient of receiving a related kidney, one must place the negative reaction of a few donors and families and the small physical risk to the donor. It should be noted that the alternatives to related donation are not without psychological stress. A minority of cadaver donor families also experience negative reactions to the donation. Furthermore, if the recipient dies, as he has been more likely to do after a cadaver donation, the stress for the grieving family and for relatives who may have been willing to donate could exceed that of the few negative related donors.

244 ROBERTA G. SIMMONS

In the final analysis, the decision concerning related donors is an ethical, not an empirical, one. Which costs and which sources of stress should be absorbed and which should not be tolerated are matters of policy not science. However, it is our impression that certain sources of stresses are more visible to the policy-making physicians than others. A physical complication for a related donor and a psychological negative reaction on the part of a related donor tend to be very visible and to impact with great drama on the medical staff, who continue to care for the recipient over the long term. On the other hand, the long-term *positive* reactions of most related donors are not seen by the physicians. Also, physicians are unaware of problems among cadaver donor families whom they almost never see after the transplant. Similarly, if a patient dies after a cadaver transplant, the grief of the surviving blood relatives, while assumed, is not likely to remain in view for any length of time.

A few caveats are in order concerning our findings. It is possible that donors at the University of Minnesota react more positively than those in other parts of the country and in other programs. The ethnic background of these Midwestern donors and the optimism of the medical staff associated with this program may have a favorable effect. (However, studies by Fellner and Marshall,[12,13] and Eisendrath, Guttman, and Murray,[21] are compatible with ours.)

Other qualifications to our conclusions are also relevant. Cognitive dissonance may be operative; many related donors may be unwilling to evaluate such a personal sacrifice negatively. More important, the measures used in this study made donation salient. It is unclear whether the donors would have appeared infused with as high self-esteem and great feelings of well-being if they were measured by a questionnaire in a setting that did not make their donation salient—if they were unaware that the person measuring them knew of the donation. Nevertheless, the reaction of these donors in this program when donation is made salient appears to be positive, by and large. Certainly the burden of proof would appear to rest on individuals who claim that related donation should be curtailed because of widespread negative psychological effects and unwillingness to donate.[4]

As part of the analysis here, we have identified types of donors who react more postively to the donation and types who have reacted more negatively. No factor is a good enough predictor for us to recommend halting the use of one type of relative as donor. However, since ambivalence prior to donation is correlated with long-term negative feelings, more screening for ambivalence and elimination of the few extremely ambivalent donors would seem advisable. Counselling help for other relatives who wish to donate despite normal fears would also be beneficial.

REFERENCES

1. SOMMERS, B. G., SUTHERLAND, D. E. R., SIMMONS, R. L., HOWARD, R. J., and NAJARIAN, J. S. Prognosis after renal transplantation: cumulative influence of combined risk factors. *Transplantation*, 1979, *27*, 4–7.

2. LARGIADÈR, F. Transplant organ procurement and preservation. *Documents geigy transplants: the way ahead*, CIBA-GEIGY Limited, 1971, pp. 3–5.

3. BREWER, S. P. Donors of organs seen as victims. *New York Times*, April 19, 1970, 36.

4. KATZ, J. and CAPRON, A. M. *Catastrophic diseases: who decides what?* New York: Russell Sage Foundation, 1975.

5. HAMBURGER, J. and CROSNIER, J. Moral and ethical problems in transplantation. In F. Rapaport and J. Dausset (Eds.), *Human transplantation*. New York: Grune and Stratton, 1968.

6. SPANOS, P. K., SIMMONS, R. L., LAMPE, E., RATTAZZI, L. C., KJELLSTRAND, C. M., GOETZ, F. C., and NAJARIAN, J. S. Complications of related kidney donation. *Surgery*, 1974, *76*, 741–747.

7. SIMMONS, R. G., KLEIN, S. D., and SIMMONS, R. L. *Gift of life: the social and psychological impact of organ transplantation*. New York: Wiley Interscience, 1977.

8. SIMMONS, R. G. Related donors: costs and gains. *Transplantation Proceedings*, 1977, *9*, 143–145.

9. SIMMONS, R. G., and KAMSTRA-HENNEN, L. The living related kidney donor: psychological reactions when the kidney fails. *Dialysis and Transplantation*, 1979, *8*, 572–574.

10. ROSENBERG, M. *Society and the adolescent self-image*. Princeton, NJ: Princeton University Press, 1965.

11. SIMMONS, R. G., KLEIN, S. D., and THORNTON, K. The family member's decision to be a kidney transplant donor. *Journal of Comparative Family Studies*, 1973, *4*, 88–115.

12. FELLNER, C. H., and MARSHALL, J. R. Twelve kidney donors. *Journal of the American Medical Association*, 1968, *206*, 2703–2707.

13. FELLNER, C. H., and MARSHALL, J. R. Kidney donors: the myth of informed consent. *American Journal of Psychiatry*, 1970, *126*, 1245–1251.

14. KAMSTRA-HENNEN, L., and SIMMONS, R. G. Ethics of related donation: The unsuccessful case. *Proceedings of the Clinical Dialysis and Transplantation Forum*, 1979, *8*.

15. CRAMOND, W. A. Renal homotransplantation: some observations on recipients and donors. *British Journal of Psychiatry*, 1967, *113*, 1223–1230.

16. LITMAN, T. The family as a basic unit in health and medical care: a social behavioral overview. *Social Science and Medicine*, 1974, *8*, 495–519.

17. RAPAPORT, F. T. *A second look at life: transplantation and dialysis patients: their own stories.* New York: Grune and Stratton, 1973.

18. BERNSTEIN, D. M. and SIMMONS, R. G. The adolescent kidney donor: the right to give. *American Journal of Psychiatry*, 1974, *131*, 1338–1343.

19. SPANOS, P. K., SIMMONS, R. L., SIMMONS, R. G., GOLDBERG, M., and NAJARIAN, J. S. The aging related kidney donor: prognosis for donor, recipient and kidney. *Abstracts of the Sixth Annual Meeting of The American Society of Nephrology*, 1973.

20. FULTON, J., FULTON, R., and SIMMONS, R. The cadaver donor and the gift of life. In R. G. Simmons, S. D. Klein, and R. L. Simmons, *Gift of life: the social and psychological impact of organ transplantation*. New York: Wiley Interscience, 1977.

21. EISENDRATH, R. M., GUTTMAN, R. D., and MURRAY, J. E. Psychological considerations in the selection of kidney transplant donors. *Surgery, Gynecology, and Obstetrics* 1969, *129*, 243–248.

22. SIMMONS, R. G., BRUCE, J., BIENVENUE, R., and FULTON, J. Who signs an organ donor card: traditionalism versus transplantation. *Journal of Chronic Diseases*, 1974, *27*, 491–502.

23. BRADBURN, N. M. *The structure of psychological well-being*. Chicago: Aldine, 1969.

22
Stopping Immunosuppressant Therapy Following Successful Renal Transplantation
Two-Year Follow-Up

STEPHEN ARMSTRONG, KEITH JOHNSON, AND
JEANNE HOPKINS

Most transplant physicians assume that immunosuppression must be carried out indefinitely for all renal transplant recipients, except for patients who receive transplant from an identical twin. When transplant recipients stop immunosuppression voluntarily, which happens relatively infrequently,[1] their behavior certainly threatens both the renal graft and their life.[2,3] The irrationality of voluntary cessation of immunosuppression calls for some explanation.

This purposeful and odd behavior can be explained psychodynamically. The transplanted organ can activate unconscious fantasies, hostile introjects, and malevolent thinking which is not reality oriented or "neutralized" thinking.[4,5] Under the stress of surgery and postoperative recovery, the patient experiences "the stress of the situation in terms of primary process and deals with the transplant experience in fantastic, primitive, and instinct-laden terms."[5a] A patient may fear, for example, having stolen the donated kidney, or having accidentally acquired the donor's traits, which may not be ones he wanted. The patient also can fear the organ's potential to damage him, or enslavement to the doctors or

STEPHEN ARMSTRONG, PH.D. • Assistant Clinical Professor, Tufts University School of Medicine; Associate in Psychiatry, University of Massachusetts School of Medicine; and Adjunct Assistant Professor, University of Massachusetts School of Public Health, Springfield, Massachusetts.   KEITH JOHNSON, M.D. • Assistant Professor of Medicine, Division of Nephrology, Vanderbilt University School of Medicine; and Co-Director Nashville Transplant Program, Nashville, Tennessee.   JEANNE HOPKINS, R.N. • Transplant Nurse Coordinator, Nashville Transplant Service, Vanderbilt Hospital, Nashville, Tennessee.

donor.[6,7] The new kidney also changes family relations[8,9] and other psychological functions.[10] This psychodynamic explanation proposes that, by rejecting the transplant, the patient preserves his bodily integrity, represses his conflict, and restores equilibrium to his family and himself.

This type of explanation may fit other forms of odd behavior in other types of transplantation[10]; it is the only plausible explanation that has received attention in the psychological and psychiatric literature. Our research team has followed ten patients for two years after they had voluntarily stopped immunosuppression following successful transplantation, trying to understand such unusual behavior as much as the theory and our clinical practice allow.

METHOD

Study 1*

In 1976, three months to three years postcessation, we asked five surviving patients to have a psychiatric diagnostic and assessment interview. This interview included questions predicted by the intrapsychic stress theory, such as their family relations before and after the transplant, fantasies about hemodialysis, transplantation, the donor, the newly acquired or lost transplant, reactions to the surgery and to immunosuppression, other fears, and so forth. We sought collateral information by telephone or personal interviews with an in-house member of the patient's family, from the medical record, and by concurrent physical examination. The five patients also completed a MMPI and Rorschach testing.[11] We compiled as much information on a sixth, deceased patient as we could from records and collateral interview.

Study 2†

In 1978 we asked the same five surviving patients to continue the study and we sought further information from five new patients who, in the intervening two years, had decided to stop immunosuppression. Additionally, we added a small sample of patients who had involuntarily rejected a kidney transplant because of medical reasons. We also added a

*Study 1 was conducted while Stephen Armstrong was a NIMH Postdoctoral Fellow in Clinical Psychology 1 F32 MH05189-01, Vanderbilt University.
†Study 2 was supported by a small grant from the Dialysis Clinics, Inc. (a nonprofit corporation) to Stephen Armstrong.

number of measures to the second study: (1) A semistructured standard psychiatric interview (SSIAM) that has been used as a baseline measure for psychotherapy studies.[12,13] We asked the same questions regarding the patient's fantasies and introjects, beliefs about the kidney, and their family relations that had been asked in Study 1; (2) A standard measure of external social stress that has been used in a number of studies of medically and psychosomatically ill patients (Social Readjustment Rating Scale—SRRS)[14–17]; (3) A standard 53-item psychiatric and somatic symptom inventory completed by the patient (Brief Symptom Inventory-BSI)[18–20]; (4) Rorschach testing[11]; with (5) Mayman's object relations modification of the Rorschach inquiry,[21] and with Klopfer's prognostic rating scale.[22,23] The investigators also studied the patient's medical records. Patients donated their interview time, which was about two hours; all patients are volunteers without promises or inducements and with informed consent.

FINDINGS

The number of patients having stopped immunosuppression is small (11 cases in the series of 460 Nashville transplants). Hence, we can make statements only by stating our "clinical impression," and by comparing the small numbers of patients who voluntarily stop immunosuppression to the normative standards of psychological health established in other studies of medically ill patients. One complication to our study, however, is that all of our patients were medically well and without major complication at the time of cessation, interview, and follow-up, i.e., they had chronic and medically well managed conditions, not acute medical provocation. Thus, we believe that patients who stop immunosuppression do so because of psychological, not medical, complications.

One patient died soon after cessation from medical complications; the other 10 are alive. Six of the surviving patients have rejected the transplant or have had transplant failure resulting from the lack of immunosuppression. Three patients continue without loss of kidney function despite stopping. One last patient has maintained kidney function for more than three years without immunosuppression, but he surely is an exception to the general rule that posttransplant medications are required.

Cessation Episodes

These patients stop their drugs at any time after the transplant, from one month to nine years, with an average of 23 months. Doctors' and nurses' phone calls to re-engage each patient in medical treatment are not usually successful, until the patient arrives at the hospital in acute rejection crisis. Only two patients have "tempted fate" more than once by precipitating acute rejection episodes voluntarily.

Psychiatric Illness

Every patient has experienced symptoms of minor depressive disorder in the course of the medical treatment, but only one patient has a psychiatric illness, based on currently applicable research diagnostic criteria for psychiatric illness.[24] While some physicians argue informally that patients who voluntarily stop immunosuppression "must be crazy," 10 of the 11 in this patient series are not mentally ill.

Psychological Distress

Despite being free from mental illness, all patients are distressed acutely with medical and financial worries. This stress is very potent, more than that which three-quarters of a random population ever faces. This stress lasts longer in their lives, also, because of the chronicity of their condition. Yet the voluntary cessation patients also report major personal conflicts within their family or loss of an important family member. The patients who involuntarily reject their transplants report less intense intrafamilial conflicts, and this difference between groups is clinically significant. Moreover, at follow-up, both groups continue to be medically and financially stressed, but the intrafamily stress or losses have become equal over time. In short, for patients who stop their medications, the family stress "cools off" to a level approximating that of other kidney patients.

Intrapsychic Stress Theory

In the first study, nonblinded Rorschach and MMPI interpretation did not seem to support the intrapsychic stress theory: hostile introjects, malevolent imagery, oral frustrations, and perceptual disorganization scores were approximately normal for three patients, slightly elevated for one patient, and definitely elevated for the patient with concurrent psychiatric illness. Psychiatric interview questions, however, did support the notion of reactivated fantastic thinking impinging on the decision to stop immunosuppression. Our team constructed a plausible retrospective psychodynamic rationale for each patient.

Example 1. A 17-year-old, Patient A had been doing reasonably well despite his ambivalence about his father. When he grew long hair and his father cut him off, however, Patient A stopped his immunosuppression, "declaring" his independence and reenacting with the doctors his suffering with his father.

Example 2. A 21-year-old obese, dependent homosexual male, Patient B received a live-related sibling kidney, and, at the same time, moved away from mother's house. He soon undid the kidney transplant, thereby also undoing the separation from mother, her cooking, and the gift that forced him away from his family.

We also think it is psychodynamically important that nearly all voluntary cessation patients (10 of 11) have learned of their kidney disease as children or adolescents, and nearly all disclose the same ambivalence about immunosuppression that juvenile diabetics tend to have toward insulin.[25] Our immunosuppression patients are really "testing the limits" psychodynamically.

Psychological Continuities

Patients who live through an acute rejection episode because of their misplaced willfulness suffer great medical and psychological upset, even if the kidney transplant can be medically salvaged. Our patients have grown because of their suffering, and growth is confirmed on a number of measures. Rorschach prognostic and object relations measures are less primitive and anguished; thematic concerns over oral frustration, body and self boundaries, impulsivity, and untested fears are more controlled and organized. Voluntary cessation patients also find appropriate social and cultural contexts in which to function, for example, by completing their schooling, getting a job, or adopting adult expressions of developmentally earlier interests.

Rejection episodes are the darkest times of a patient's life. When asked what they would say to someone awaiting a transplant, our patients say that others should have optimism and courage about a new transplant. Every patient says he would guard a new transplant carefully. Thus, from the suffering he has endured, the voluntary cessation patient emerges with a newer, more mature sense of direction and purposefulness.

COMMENT

Whenever an event has a low probability (about 2% in the Nashville series) and indicators of its possible occurrence are not certain, one cannot "screen" a population efficiently.[26] Standardized psychological testing or psychiatric interviews, standing alone, are unlikely to identify voluntary cessation patients before the fact. High-risk patients can be identified. Transplant patients who voluntarily stop immunosuppression do not attend follow-up clinic, and unexplained absences should be investigated. They also are people who had kidney disease prior to adulthood. They also are testing the limits of their family and are struggling for a life independent of doctors or medications.

Voluntary cessation of immunosuppression can occur at any time posttransplantation. These patients are medically and psychiatrically well and are highly stressed. Voluntary cessation patients have particular family concerns, however, about loss or abandonment of special family members, or independence from their families, which may be part of maturing past adolescence. At the time of cessation, patients offer explanations consistent with major intrapsychic fluctuations, especially about hostile introjects and feelings of great guilt. When a patient destroys a kidney, family and psychological equilibrium are restored, but only at great personal cost.

Even if a patient loses a kidney through voluntary cessation of immunosuppression, however, there is a reasonable course of psychological maturation over time, due to the patient's attempts to understand his thinking about himself and the kidney and from entry into psychosocially appropriate activities. There is no psychological reason to exclude a voluntary cessation patient *a priori* from another transplantation.

REFERENCES

1. HARRINGTON, J. M.D. Personal communication, 1978.
2. ARMSTRONG, S., JOHNSON, K., and RITCHIE, R. Patients who voluntarily stop immunosuppressants following successful kidney transplantation. Paper presented at Southeastern Dialysis and Transplantation Association, Nashville, Tennessee, 1976.
3. UEHLING, D. T., HUSSEY, J. L., WEINSTEIN, A. B., WANK, R., and BACK, F. H. Cessation of immunosuppression after renal transplantation. *Surgery*, 1976, 79, 278–282.
4. BASCH, S. M. The intrapsychic integration of a new organ: a clinical study of kidney transplantation. *Psychoanalytic Quarterly*, 1973, 42, 364–384.
5. TOURKOW, L. P. Psychic consequences of loss and replacement of body parts. *American Psychoanalytic Association Journal*, 1974, 22, 170–181.
5a. CASTELNUOVO-TEDESCO, P. Organ transplant, body image, psychosis. *Psychoanalytic Quarterly*, 1973, 42, 349–363.
6. VIEDERMAN, M. Adaptive and maladaptive regression in hemodialysis. *Psychiatry*, 1974a, 37, 68–77.
7. VIEDERMAN, M. The search for meaning in renal transplantation. *Psychiatry*, 1974b, 37, 283–290.
8. KEMPH, J. P. Psychotherapy with patients receiving a kidney transplant. *American Journal of Psychiatry*, 1967, 124, 623–629.
9. KEMPH, J. P. Kidney transplant and shifts in family dynamics. *American Journal of Psychiatry*, 1969, 125, 1485–1490.

10. MUSLIN, H. L. On acquiring a kidney. *American Journal of Psychiatry*, 1971, *127*, 1185–1188.
11. EXNER, J. *The Rorschach: a comprehensive system*. New York: John Wiley, 1974.
12. GURLAND, B. J., YORKSTON, N. J., GOLDBERG, K., FLEISS, J. L., SLOANE, R. B., and CRISTOL, A. H. The structured and scaled interview to assess maladjustment (SSIAM): II. Factor analysis, reliability, and validity. *Archives of General Psychiatry*, 1972, *27*, 264–269.
13. GURLAND, B. J., YORKSTON, N. J., STONE, R., JR., FRANK, J. D., and FLEISS, J. L. The structured and scaled interview to assess maladjustment (SSIAM): I. Description, rationale, and development *Archives of General Psychiatry*, 1972, *27*, 259–263.
14. GRANT, I., GEIST, M., and YAGER, J. Scaling of life events by psychiatric patients and normals. *Journal of Psychosomatic Research*, 1976, *20*, 141–149.
15. HOLMES, T. H., and RAHE, R. H. The social readjustment rating scale. *Journal of Psychosomatic Research*, 1967, *11*, 213–218.
16. SCHLESS, A. P., TEICHMAN, A., MENDELS, J., and DiGIACOMO, J. N. The role of stress as a precipitating factor of psychiatric illness. *British Journal of Psychiatry*, 1977, *130*, 19–22.
17. VINOKUR, A., and SELZER, M. L. Desirable versus undesirable life events: their relationship to stress and mental distress. *Journal of Personality and Social Psychology*, 1975, *32*, 329–337.
18. DEROGATIS, L. R. SCL-90-R. Revised Version. Manual-I. Clinical Psychometrics Research Unit, Johns Hopkins School of Medicine, Baltimore, MD, 1977.
19. DEROGATIS, L. R., LIPMAN, R. S., and COVI, L. The SCL-90: an outpatient psychiatric rating scale, preliminary report. *Psychopharmacology Bulletin*, 1973, *9*, 13–27.
20. DEROGATIS, L. R., LIPMAN, R. S., COVI, L., and RICKELS, K. Factorial invariance of symptom dimensions in anxious and depressive neuroses. *Archives of General Psychiatry*, 1972, *27*, 659–665.
21. MAYMAN, M. Early memories and character structure. *Journal of Projective Techniques and Personality Assessment*, 1968, *32*, 303–316.
22. KLOPFER, B. Rorschach prognostic rating scale. In B. Knopfer, M.D. Ainsworth, W. G. Klopfer, and R. R. Holt (Eds.), *Developments in the Rorschach technique*, Vol.1: *technique and theory*. New York: Harcourt, Brace, and World, 1954.
23. SHEEHAN, J. G., FREDERICK, C. J., ROSEVEAR, W. H., and SPIEGELMAN, M. A validity study of the Rorschach prognostic rating scale. *Journal of Projective Techniques*, 1954, *18*, 233–239.
24. SPITZER, R. L., and ENDICOTT, J. Research diagnostic criteria (RDC) for a selected group of functional disorders. Biometrics Research, New York Psychiatric Institute, 722 West 168th Street, New York, N.Y. 10032.
25. HOLTZMAN, J. M.D. Personal communication, 1978.
26. MEEHL, P., and ROSEN, A. Antecedent probability and the efficiency of psychometric signs, patterns, or cutting scores. *Psychological Bulletin*, 1955, *52*, 194–216.

23
Consultation–Liaison in a Renal Transplant Unit

HELLMUTH FREYBERGER

INTRODUCTION

Consultation–liaison in the renal transplant unit at Hannover Medical School began in Summer, 1976, and has developed up to now, step by step, in a somewhat experimental way. We emphasize this experimental building-up way because, to the best of our knowledge, there has not existed up to now a consultation–liaison unit which could serve as a model for us. Concerning the number of patients transplanted, initially, in 1975, 35 patients and in 1977, 100 patients underwent this procedure which was done by the Abdominal and Transplant-Surgery Department of our medical school. Our consultation–liaison activity was performed by our patient care, our regular conferences with participation of the nurses and psychosomaticist, and our teaching.

PATIENT CARE

Consultation–liaison with regard to patient care included the following four activities:

1. Group therapy sessions in the renal transplant inpatient unit
2. Informal inpatient visits by the psychosomaticist
3. The psychosomaticist's consultations with the surgeons
4. Psychotherapeutic interventions with individual patients.

HELLMUTH FREYBERGER, M.D. • Professor of Psychosomatics, University of Hannover Medical School, Hannover-Kleefeld, German Federal Republic.

Group Sessions in the Renal Transplant Inpatient Unit

A group therapy session with inpatients for a period of one-and-a-half hours takes place every three weeks in the inpatient unit. The number of patients participating is usually between five and eight, in addition to two nurses. These sessions often result in the following three potentially therapeutic activities.

First, it permits the patient to verbalize and thus by catharsis results in some patients gaining symptomatic relief. In addition, as the consequence of the perception that other persons are suffering from similar problems, patients will often be more accepting of their own problems. In the patients' view, the major emotional problems surround the question of the success or rejection of the kidney transplant. Patients often verbalize the following two themes:

1. In the view of a threatened transplant rejection, the patient feels he is "sitting on a powder keg"; he can be compared to a person who is living in fear of an earthquake. Furthermore, we observed in these patients labile self-esteem, depression, and anxiety. The therapist, in a sense, gives permission to the patient for the ventilation of these impairing affects.
2. The patient often has hostile feelings as the result of real, threatening, or fantasied frustrations as a result of his contact with nurses, nephrologists, and surgeons. We regard it as essential that the therapist perceives the patient's manifest or underlying frustration/aggressive feelings so that he can allow the patient to express them.

Second, group sessions permit the facilitation of the mutual evaluation of medical problems so that the patient becomes an "expert" with regard to his disease and its treatment. If this aim can be realized, the patient is often better prepared to cooperate with the surgeons and nurses caring for him.

Third, group sessions usually result in dealing with patients' denial. Denial is the most frequent defense mechanism used by patients in the renal transplant unit. Denial is particularly evident in early transplant situations when anxiety, depression, and weakened self-esteem are often at their greatest intensity. We differentiate the following three degrees of intensity of denial.[1,2]

1. Realistically adapted denial which occurs in the majority of the patients and is connected with a sufficient introspective ability concerning the acceptance of the disease situation and the understanding of the therapeutic measures.

2. Highly intensive denial which is connected with a lack of self-reflective ability. Here the patient shows a partial or almost complete withdrawal of his self-reflective ability with regard to the disease and therapy situation.
3. Insufficient denial which is also connected with a lack of a self-reflective ability as the consequence of the overflowing of the patient's psychic apparatus with painful emotions. Simultaneously, highly increased oral–narcissistic needs are evident in the patient.

Inpatients treated in renal transplant units have denial in a realistically adapted way only insofar as the denial is not too marked. The denial must leave a certain amount of the patient's intrapsychic capacity for reality intact so that he is able to perceive and sufficiently control his outside needs and emotions. Only then is there a healthy reconciliation with the demands of the therapy program. Here, reactive depression, anxiety, and weakened self-esteem are functioning in the sense of a "signal function" with regard to acceptance of the disease and therapeutic measures. In this case of realistically adapted denial, these reactive responses are often moderately pronounced and usually can be tolerated by the patient without decompensation. Consequently, the patient is usually very cooperative and is able to accept the therapeutic measures. This "signal function" which represents one of the characteristics of the reactive responses, is lost in patients experiencing highly intensive and insufficient denial. The highly intensive denial results in a nearly total repudiation of the disease situation and the understanding of its treatment. In the case of insufficient denial, the patient tends to overly fear the disease and its treatment with the consequence of relapsing states of death anxieties and/or hopelessness. Simultaneously, highly increased oral–narcissistic needs occur in this patient. Let me clarify these three degrees of intensity denial on the basis of the patient's experience following the kidney transplant rejection.

If the transplanted kidney is finally rejected, then the patient with realistically adapted denial experiences this event as a major trauma, often followed by transient states of mild hopelessness. However, the patient's self-reflective ability with regard to the disease situation and therapeutic necessity is not lost. The most profound degree of hopelessness is evident at the occasion of the surgeon's decision to remove the transplanted kidney. Fortunately, because of their ability to use denial, these patients are soon able to reduce the painful emotions following their severe loss and to reflect about this serious crisis. Following the nephrectomy the patient tends to become emotionally stabilized and looks forward to the possibility of a second transplantation. Most people are interested in receiving a new kidney transplant as soon as possible.

When the patient with highly intensive denial experiences transplant rejection, because of his lack of self-reflective ability, he is usually not sufficiently prepared for this severe crisis. He may repress the dysphoric affects associated with this event and refuse to accept the appropriate therapy and/or he may express the wish to leave the hospital. In a minority of the highly intensive deniers, their very rigid defenses can break down and they may experience relapsing states of death anxiety and/or hopelessness which is more pronounced than in patients with realistically adapted denial.

Insufficient deniers often experience the same degree of difficulty as the high-intensity deniers with transplant rejection. Both groups may experience severe death anxieties and depression including considerable hopelessness. Both groups are usually not prepared to emotionally master this severe loss. In our group sessions the possibility of a second renal transplantation induced no encouragement or support for the insufficient or high-intensity deniers, in fact most refused a future procedure.

Concerning dealing with the renal transplant patients' denial during the group sessions, the therapist carefully observed whether or not a realistically adapted denial has occurred in individual patients. In the case of realistically adapted denial, the therapist should support appropriate behavior modalities. However, in the case of highly intensive denial, the patient's too strong defense may be weakened by encouraging him to verbalize his denied thoughts and feelings. In the case of insufficient denial, the patient's oral–narcissistic needs should be partly satisfied by the therapist's support, and if necessary by individual sessions.

The Informal Inpatients' Visits by the Psychosomaticist

The psychosomaticist made short visits to each patient three times weekly as a result of learning the emotional difficulties of patients during the group sessions and as a consequence of conversations with the surgeons and nurses. The particular aim of these visits was to identify those patients who showed traits of highly intensive or insufficient denial. Both for consultation and teaching it was also very useful for the psychosomaticist to have regular contact with the surgeons and nurses in order to discuss patients' medical courses and emotional adaptation.

The Psychosomaticist's Consultations with the Surgeons

The psychosomaticist participated in consulations with the surgeons once weekly, which involved the following:

1. The patients' psychosocial problems and discussion of possible psychotherapeutic maneuvers.
2. Those dialysis patients who are very ambivalent concerning renal transplantation. Methods of positively motivating these patients are discussed.
3. Dealing with related donors about their relationship with the potential recipient. The necessity for these discussions arises as a result of ambivalence within the donor–recipient relationship. The nature of the donor's motivation is discussed including the clarification of the donor's motivation. Such motivation may be based on altruism and/or founded on neurotic acting-out and/or a result of guilt feelings as the consequence of the relatives' pressure. We eventually decide if the relative's donation is realistically adapted or if it is necessary to treat psychotherapeutically the donor's defended hostility and guilt feelings.

Psychotherapeutic Interventions with Individual Patients

Psychotherapeutic interventions concerned inpatients and outpatients who were in need of a special psychosomaticist–patient relationship. Although nurses and surgeons are often engaged in the solving of the patient's problems, the psychosomaticist is available if they are not able to cope with the patient. The psychotherapeutic technique which is usually applied in transplant patients can be described by the term "supportive psychotherapy." It often involves the stabilization of patient's denial on the basis of some satisfaction of the patient's oral–narcissistic needs and in realistically adapted denial, acceptance of the disease process, and therapeutic measures. Supportive psychotherapeutical techniques usually involve the following six steps:

1. Developing a stable object relationship by regular visits of the psychosomaticist which concentrate on the patient's emotional needs.
2. Consistent availability of the psychosomaticist. This availability satisfies oral–narcissistic needs while building an object relationship. Questions are answered and advice is given.
3. Permitting the patient to verbalize his unpleasant emotions. The therapist in a sense gives permission to the patient for the ventilation of his displeasure which provides emotional relief.
4. The confrontation of the patient's tendency for oral–narcissistic acting-out. It is important to help the patient come to terms with his oral–narcissistic state. His acting-out around this drive should be minimized.

5. Psychological handling of medical procedure and equipment. Patients treated in renal transplant units develop positive feelings about objects and people that help produce good effects, such as life-saving equipment as well as surgeons and nurses. This response is a defense against anxiety. It is often one of the tasks of the psychosomaticist to strengthen this defense.
6. Dealing with current conflictual situations. If there are evident conflictual situations, confrontation and interpretations are often therapeutic.

The following three variants of supportive psychotherapy are necessary if the patients show evidence of highly intensive or insufficient denial.

a. In the case of highly intensive denial, the patient can totally repress his emotional pain and/or refuse to accept appropriate diagnostic procedures and even therapy. Here, the patient often shows no motivation for dealing with psychological problems. Therefore, to establish a stable object-relationship leading to catharsis we arrange a 45-minute interview. The personal presence of the psychosomaticist, and his continuous verbal support, is often decisive. This informal interview tends to weaken the patient's defense of denial and also motivates the patient to verbalize his denied emotional pain. At times the patient cautiously confronts his denial.

b. When the patient's denial is insufficient with consequent states of death anxiety and hopelessness, the following two psychotherapeutic interventions are advised.[3]

First, manifest death anxieties can be reduced by encouraging catharsis—by interpreting those unconscious or preconscious factors which cause the anxiety. After the catharsis—and not before—we support the patient and even give him advice.

Second, in states of severe hopelessness the psychosomaticist affirms his understanding of the patient's greatly impaired emotional state as the consequence of his critical illness. Furthermore, the therapist has to construct supportive and encouraging remarks on the basis of the patient's spontaneous verbalizations. However, the mere presence of the psychosomaticist is often sufficient in itself to achieve a gradual improvement in the patient's outlook.

c. When these psychotherapeutic techniques fail to affect the patient's denial, close relatives should be called upon to provide emotional support for the patient and, at times, help produce possible mutual confrontations.

The indications for psychotherapy in transplant patients may be viewed as follows: (1) when the patient demonstrates marked traits of highly intensive or insufficient denial, and (2) when the patient has a highly conflictual situation.

Starting from these indications, the reason for the frequency of psychotherapeutic interventions were the following:

1. In 16 inpatients and 4 outpatients who were suffering from strong depressive and anxiety feelings and severe weakened self-esteem precipitated by threatening or actual transplant rejection, the resumption of dialysis represented a particular intensive emotional trauma. The patients simultaneously manifested insufficient denial.
2. In 5 inpatients and 1 outpatient, because of highly intensive denial and consequently reduced cooperativeness.
3. In 2 inpatients and 4 outpatients, dealing with present conflict situations between patients and their relatives.
4. In 2 inpatients and 2 outpatients, psychotherapy of the relative because of episodic or relapsing states of discouragement.
5. In 2 outpatients because of difficulty adhering to their diet.

These supportive psychotherapeutic interventions may be carried out by students working as auxiliary therapists if they are continuously supervised. In our medical school, students serving in the Psychosomatic Department may be called upon to serve in such a capacity with medical and surgical patients.

The duration of psychotherapy was 1–10 sessions in 30 patients. In four patients there were occasional sessions and/or phone contacts. With regard to the phone contacts, we were very impressed with the high supportive psychotherapeutic effectiveness of these contacts. It is our belief that phone contacts may be both markedly time-saving and have far-reaching psychotherapeutic value.

REGULAR CONFERENCES OF NURSES WITH THE PSYCHOSOMATICIST

These conferences took place every four weeks for a period of one-and-a-half hours with five to seven nurses. The conferences provide a forum for discussion of patients and of the stresses of the professional team. The staff's problems are undertaken as related to highly intensive or insufficient deniers as well as staff reactions to transplant rejection, reactions to hostile patients, and many other issues related to patient care. These conferences have the structure of a Balint Group, namely, the reflections of the group about a case history, which is given by a nurse who is having problems with a patient. The associations of the nurses are given and the interpretations of this group process are made by the psychosomaticist. A group of dynamic process comes into action which not only allows psychological insight with regard to individual members but also clarifies the patient's problems. In the view of the nurses, their greatest stresses occur in dealing with the following four groups of patients:

1. The highly intensive deniers.
2. Those insufficient deniers who show marked hostility feelings following transplant rejection.
3. Those patients with transplant rejection who received their kidneys from a live donor.
4. Patients with suicidal danger following the threat or actual transplant rejection.

TEACHING

Our consultation–liaison activities with regard to teaching include the following three activities:

1. The nurses' presence in the group sessions.
2. The psychosomaticist's regular contacts with the surgeons and nurses following the informal inpatient's visits. These teaching activities bring with it considerable advanced training effects.
3. The Balint Group activities with students working as auxiliary therapists.

CONCLUSIONS

These various consultation–liaison activities, which have been described above, found a realization in the Hannover Department of Abdominal and Transplant Surgery. Recently, Lipowski wrote, ". . . that one who has worked as a liaison psychiatrist for more than 10 years is considered a 'grizzled veteran.' " I was intensively engaged in liaison psychiatric activity in internal medicine for 12 years, and thus became a "semigrizzled veteran." However, on the basis of my three years in dealing with the Hannover surgeons and nurses my "semigrizzled veteran" condition was lessened. I felt much more satisfaction with regard to consultation–liaison with surgery. This was a consequence of my acceptance by the surgeons and nurses as a function of the openmindedness of Hannover's Department of Surgery. Also, my greater satisfaction was the consequence of the contrasting views of the internists from the surgeons with regard to liaison. The internist may perceive the psychosomaticist as a competitor with regard to patient care, teaching, and research. Internists can react with an insecurity associated with the danger of loss of their professional identity. In contrast, according to my observations, the surgeon does not experience the psychosomaticist as a competitor. Furthermore, I have experienced that usually the surgeon tends to accept the psychosomaticist's opinion more fully than the internist's. Discussions with the internist concerning diagnostic and therapeutic problems in patient care practically never occur in my contacts with the surgeons. In addition, my greater satisfaction concerning consultation–liaison activity in surgery may have been influenced by the different atmospheres of the dialysis center as a special unit of medicine on the one hand, and the renal transplant center as a special unit of surgery, on the other hand. According to my long-term observations, the atmosphere of the dialysis unit with the unchanging outpatient group can be a "subdepressive monotonous climate." Dialysis nurses remain "calm" and dependent. In contrast, the transplant unit is an inpatient service in which patients have a relatively short stay. Here, the nurses show some similarity to those who are working in critical-care nursing, namely, they are more likely to be aggressive and self-assertive because they are taught to make critical decisions rapidly. The climate of the transplant unit, in my view, is more emotionally gratifying and the relationship to the patient more stimulating and happy, even with the patient feeling he is "sitting on a powder keg" because of the potentially threatened transplant rejection. The two patient groups can be described by the following statements: In the view of the dialysis patient, part of his normal life is coming to an end and in the view of the transplant patient a new life is beginning. Eisendrath's conclusion is correct that, "in most cases, a successful kidney transplant is the best psychotherapy for anyone in chronic end-stage of renal failure."[5]

REFERENCES

1. NEMIAH, J., FREYBERGER, H., SIFNEOS, P. E. Alexithymia, a view of the psychosomatic process. In O. W. Hill (Ed.), *Recent advances in psychosomatic medicine*. London: Butterworths, 1976.
2. FREYBERGER, H. Supportive psychotherapeutic techniques in primary and secondary alexithymia. *Psychotherapy and Psychosom.* 1977, *28*, 337–342.
3. FREYBERGER, H. Psychosomatic aspects of an intensive care unit. In J. G. Howells (Ed.), *Modern perspectives in the psychiatric aspect of surgery*. New York: Brunner/Mazel, 1976.
4. LIPOWSKI, Z. J. Consultation–liaison psychiatry: past, present and future. In R. O. Pasnau (Ed.), *Consultation–liaison psychiatry*. New York: Grune and Stratton, 1975, pp. 1–28.
5. EISENDRATH, R. M. Adaptation to renal transplantation. In J. G. Howells (Ed.), *Modern perspectives in the psychiatric aspects of surgery*. New York: Brunner/Mazel, 1976.
6. FREYBERGER, H. Students working as auxiliary therapists with groups of psychosomatic and organically ill patients. *Bibliotheca Psychiatrica* 1978, *159*, 88–113.

24
Psychotherapeutic Intervention in the Kidney Transplant Service

Denton C. Buchanan

Introduction

Recent reviews of the psychological complications of kidney transplantation[1,2] have discussed a number of reactions in recipients, donors, and the family members of each. To meet these social and psychological repercussions many mental health disciplines have provided their expertise over the past decade. A liaison approach in which the mental health specialist works closely with the transplant service has provided a helpful framework for alleviating emotional distress from which both patient and health care personnel have benefited. For example, Collins[3] reported improved staff morale and reduced nurse turnover with a liaison approach utilizing a psychiatrist, psychologist, and social worker. There is little question that intervention into these psychological problems has markedly improved the quality of care since Kemph[4,5] first brought them to our attention.

Little attention has been paid to the direct role of transplant service personnel (surgeons, nephrologists, nurses, and dieticians) in meeting the emotional needs of patients. Indeed, the transplant service seldom view themselves as engaged in psychotherapeutic activities. Yet, if one analyzes the interaction between patient and staff it is clear that the transactions have psychotherapeutic intent or at least potential. For example, emotional reactions in transplant recipients tend to mimic the physiological status of the kidney. Depression typically occurs during rejection episodes, and this is a time when the treatment staff are more actively involved with the patient. The patient looks for assistance and the staff are in the best position to offer advice. This is true of psychological as well as physical issues.

Denton C. Buchanan, Ph.D. • Director of Psychology, Royal Ottawa Regional Rehabilitation Center, and Associate Professor of Medicine, University of Ottawa, Ottawa, Canada.

The major purpose of this chapter is to outline two complementary psychotherapeutic techniques that can be utilized easily and efficiently by the transplant service. The first, group psychotherapy, relies heavily upon principles of patient education, an existing function of most transplant services. The second, brief psychotherapy, discusses aspects of the patient's presentation and the causes of his emotional state, primarily depression.

In advocating the involvement of the transplant service in psychotherapy, there is no intent to diminish or replace the function of the mental health consultant or liaison person. To the contrary, the effectiveness of the mental health specialist will be extended through the involvement of the entire transplant service. As Milne[1] has stated: ". . . there is certainly a place for mental health professionals in the renal unit, but their contribution is no substitute for the concern and sensitive approach to patients and their families by every member of the transplant team."

TWO-PHASE MODEL OF GROUP PSYCHOTHERAPY

Most transplant programs in the United States have patient education components. The influence of patient education upon favorable postoperative recovery from a variety of surgical procedures has become increasingly recognized by professionals. A study by Healy[6] found that patients who received clear instructions on their surgical care were discharged three to four days earlier than noninstructed controls and had fewer physical complications. Similarly, Lindeman and Van Aerman[7] found that preoperative instructions influenced ventilatory function and provided a shorter hospital stay than patients who had not received the instruction. Similarly, Egbert[8] found that patients who received education utilized fewer narcotics and had shorter hospital stays than did control group patients. These few representative studies demonstrate the value of patient education in posttransplant physical recovery. Even greater benefit may derive from group educational efforts. Educational material about renal transplantation can be presented within a group format such that patients and family have an opportunity to discuss the material presented, interact with one another over a topic, and mutually utilize the information gained to reduce anxiety and alter behavior. Anxiety reduction occurs within the group setting when the participants have the opportunity to express their apprehensions, hear the experiences of others with similar concerns, and ventilate their anger. These emotional issues interfere with both patient well-being and the educational process. Thus, physically ill patients have been shown to acquire more information about their disease and retain it longer when the information was presented in a group rather than individually.[9]

The use of group discussions for physically ill patients dates back to the turn of the century[10]; however, the therapeutic benefit derived from such meetings has been questioned. Pattison, Rhodes, and Dudley[11] reported that 7 out of 12 patients with severe chronic lung disease found the discussion of the emotional aspects of their illness so threatening that they subsequently withdrew from the program. With spouses of hemodialysis patients, Shambaugh and Kanter[12] found that group discussions resulted in "the members progressively increasing sense of emotional separateness from their partners." Similarly, Ford and Long[13] described their experience with group psychotherapy for somaticizing patients and concluded that "our treatment results, however, appear more modest than those reported by some."

Other workers have been enthusiastic about the usefulness of group meetings to meet the emotional needs of a wide variety of physically ill populations including hemodialysis and renal transplant patients. Buchanan[14] has outlined the dynamics of a short-term, open-membership group discussion program for kidney transplant recipients and described positive results, at least as defined by patients' opinions. Hollon[15] has described a beneficial program utilizing a systems approach in which the entire treatment staff becomes involved with both patient and family to discuss mutual problems: "The patients and family members seem to derive true benefit from sharing experiences with others, ventilating to one another pent-up feelings, and actually 'teaching' one another how to cope. . . ." Similarly, Hartings, Pavlou, and Davis,[16] with multiple sclerosis patients, have reported encouraging results with a group approach. Suffice it to say, there is a controversy in the clinical literature over the usefulness of group discussion.

A review of various articles on this topic demonstrates an interesting divergence in the therapeutic orientations employed by successful and unsuccessful treatment programs. As a general statement, reports of unsuccessful treatment with the group approach have typically described a traditional, insight-oriented, interpretive psychiatric group format, i.e., the group leader's role was to interpret group process and to comment upon pathological behavior. Patient discussion in such groups tended to be actively directed away from their physical complaints and toward their emotional feelings. In contrast, groups that have been successful with various chronic physically ill patients have emphasized patient education, either through didactic presentation of factual material or through patient self-help. In general, these groups provided a less dynamically oriented milieu for patient participation in which discussion was encouraged without interpretation of motivation or apparent pathology. Although success is clearly a function of the goals of treatment (and certainly the goals are different in these two different styles of patient groups) it seems apparent that groups which emphasize patient education rather than the typical psychodynamically oriented group approach have proven more beneficial for chronic physically ill patients.

Patients with physical illness have some basic differences in attitude to those with emotional illness. Unlike somaticizing or psychosomatic patients, physically ill patients tend to avoid identification with their problem. The role of denial of illness in hemodialysis and transplantation has been well described and this basic defense mechanism of minimizing the disease or ignoring it outright provides a major obstacle in psychotherapeutic interaction. Consequently, insight-oriented group therapy which confronts patients with their emotional status and coping behaviors may be too threatening. A more factual presentation of basic medical and psychological aspects of transplantation reduces threat by allowing the patient to be a passive observer who may gradually personalize the topics and later become more active in the discussion.

Another reason for the apparent success of an educationally oriented group approach is that it provides an opportunity for the patients and family members to actively seek information about their disease. Buchanan[14] found that information seeking was the major activity of kidney transplant patients in a group setting. Similarly, Brock, Lawson, and Bennett[17] found a day-long education-oriented preoperative workshop for kidney transplant patients to be beneficial in the reduction of anxiety and depression. It should be noted that the early reports of group activity for the physically ill[10] effectively utilized a totally didactic orientation in helping patients cope with their illnesses.

The desire of patients to learn more about their condition can be seen in the tremendous growth of patient organized self-help clubs. Gussow and Tracy[18] investigated such organizations and found their primary purpose was to provide direct services to patients and family in the form of education about the disease, skills in management, and encouragement to deal more effectively and adaptively with their medical problem. The history of these clubs indicates a tremendous increase in the number of groups formed over the past 30 years; from 4 in 1942 to 2022 in 1972. Certainly this demonstrates the interest in the services provided.

Administration of a Two-Phase Model of Groups

The role of patient education has had a major influence in the model of group process described below. This approach to groups has been developed from experience with a number of physical illnesses[19] and attempts to combine the most therapeutic features of didactic and insight-oriented group psychotherapy. The Two-Phase Model begins with a series of meetings (approximately four) which are aimed predominantly at patient and family education. Each meeting is begun in a structured, didactic manner using films, outside speakers, and/or reading materials. A discussion period follows in which group members are encouraged to comment upon the information presented. For example, medications, the rejection process, and surgical operating room procedures are typical topics of interest. A physician may discuss in basic terms the pharmacology of medicines and why various dosages are required. A question and answer period follows in which the speaker responds to inquiries. The group leader's role is to begin to alert the members of the common interest that they have and the similarities in their concerns.

During the first four meetings many emotionally charged issues normally are raised and at that time reference is made to the following meetings that will afford an opportunity for discussing these issues at length. Generally by the fifth meeting, the group has sufficient cohesion and comfort amongst its members that they begin to discuss more personal, psychological issues. Thus, the second phase of this model has a psychological focus. During this phase the group leader continues to promote discussion by having members share their experiences on the various topics. The dynamics of this phase have been described previously.[14]

Three basic categories of participants have emerged from the Two-Phase Model. Persons who have a relatively healthy psychological adjustment to their disease and minimal emotional problems usually attend the initial education phase to attain information, but then later terminate. Approximately 25% of the participants fall in this category. Secondly, there is a larger subgroup of patients (approximately 50%) who have psychological concerns and who remain with the group in order to take advantage of all meetings. Lastly, there is another subgroup of patients (approximately 25%) who present clear adjustment problems but who apparently find the emotional discussion too threatening and either discontinue or attend erratically. It is useful therefore to start the meetings with approximately 15 members in order that 8–10 continue.

A modified intake interview usually has been utilized. The purpose has been to explain the nature of the group, to reduce the patient's anxiety, and to provide an appropriate expectation from the meetings. These interviews are supportive, nonthreatening, and emphasize the benefit to be gained. The interviews inform the group leader on the background of the patient, his experiences, strengths and weaknesses in order to utilize this information to provide support for other group members. For example, it is important for the group leader to know which participants have had previous surgery or rejections in order that their experiences may be utilized when the topic arises in the group.

A basic philosophy of the Two-Phase Model is that meetings be considered an integral part of the transplantation procedure. In keeping with this attitude, the meetings are generally held in the dialysis clinic or outpatient transplant clinic, whichever is more appropriate. Participants are familiar with the clinic and this reduces both threat and novelty to the meetings. Similarly, meetings may be held in the offices of the local chapter of the National Kidney Association. Again, this promotes the sense of "universality" of the members.

Long-term group meetings have been avoided. Generally the members have been requested to attend a complete program, usually 10 to 15 meetings, held from one to one-and-a-half hours every week or perhaps biweekly. Open membership groups have been conducted[14] in which the participants attended whenever they happened to come to the medical clinic. In general, however, a closed group for a short time (10 meetings) has proved to be more beneficial.

BRIEF PSYCHOTHERAPY

While the Two-Phase Model group seems to offer the most benefit to the most patients on a cost-efficient basis, it certainly is not intended to provide a panacea for mental ills. In fact, the group meetings often uncover underlying emotional currents that have been hidden from the transplant staff's view. This should not be considered a detriment to the program; to the contrary, it allows for the recognition of emotional concerns at an earlier stage than would otherwise happen. These emotional reactions can usually be treated with individual brief psychotherapy by the transplant staff.

Brief or short-term psychotherapy (in this context) refers to a supportive, psychologically oriented discussion that can coincide with treatment of coexisting organic problems, where needed. By definition, such therapy is time limited, usually 10 sessions or less, lasting from 15 to 30 minutes each. This time restriction avoids excessive time obligations on the treatment staff, insures that the discussion will be focused upon relevant problems, and gives the therapist a sense of security by limiting the opportunity to get involved beyond his capabilities. The issue of competence in therapy is often raised by nonpsychologically trained individuals as a reason to avoid therapy. Actually, in brief psychotherapy, much can be accomplished by utilizing the common sense of daily life combined with a sensitive and understanding attitude. Interpersonal skills are generally highly developed in treatment staff; confidence in their own abilities is all that is required. Brief supportive psychotherapy is useful, however, only for milder emotional disturbance; reactions to current stressful life events. Major problems such as organic brain syndromes, psychoses, character disorders, drug addictions, and chronic unstable personalities should not be approached in this manner.

In a recent review of the transplant literature, Abram and Buchanan[2] concluded that there were fewer psychopathological reactions following renal transplantation than in hemodialysis. The most common psychological problem was depression. Penn,[20] in a large series of 292 transplant patients, found that 32% showed postoperative depression and that seven of these patients committed suicide. Similarly, Abram, Moore, and Westervelt[21] have shown that suicide can be a significant cause of death, particularly if the transplanted organ is rejected and the patient is placed back into a dialysis program. Kemph,[22] as well as other workers, has also commented upon the depression that typically accompanies rejection episodes. As depressive reactions usually are responsive to intervention through brief psychotherapy, this section intends to assist the staff in recognizing depression, understanding the depressed patients' perspective, as well as to suggest some basic interaction techniques which allow the patient to achieve a more positive and hopeful view of himself.

Recognition of Depression

While recognition of depression may seem to be elementary, in actual fact it proves to be a much more difficult task. One cannot rely upon patients to voluntarily report their emotional distress as they are often not aware of their own depression. Those patients who do perceive their lowered mood are frequently so guilty or disappointed in themselves that they avoid spontaneously presenting the fact to the treatment staff.

Depression really represents a group of illnesses that have some features and symptoms in common. Consequently, depression may be manifested in a wide variety of ways, and not all patients have the same presenting symptomology. Some will emphasize the affective features, some the thought content or cognitive components, and others will present primarily physical complaints or "depressive equivalents."

One salient feature of depressed individuals is lowered mood or affect. There is a feeling of sadness, gloom, and despair. The aspects of life that normally give pleasure become indifferent, and there is a failure to see events in any pleasurable way. They may smile slightly at someone else's humor but be unable to see any of their own. Apathy and a sense of hopelessness pervade their mood. Anger also may be prominent. The anger can be directed outwardly at others causing the patient to react in an irritable fashion or be directed inwardly causing self-abuse and self-recrimination. Suicide, of course, is the ultimate form of self-abuse.

A second defining component of the depressed patients is the general thought pattern. They tend to be preoccupied with themselves and worried about their plight. They will ruminate about their past actions, particuarly failures, and imagine magical solutions to their present problems. That such illogical solutions do not happen to solve their problems only serves to prove the futility of their position. The topics which are not present in thought are as significant as those with which the patient is preoccupied. Past successes, jobs, pleasures, skills, and rewards are forgotten. Depressed individuals are preoccupied with their internal world and, consequently, do not attent to external issues. Thus, they often complain of "memory" problems and forgetfulness.

The patient's general behavior may be a clue for the treatment team. Depressed people tend to be slow in their movements and responses to questions. Intentional and purposeful behavior is usually diminished even if agitation and hyperactivity is apparent at first glance. Pacing the floor and wringing one's hands may give the impression of activity, but in essence they are futile, purposeless behaviors. Withdrawal from social contact and activities may be an early clue. Depressed transplant patients will often sit alone in the clinic waiting room, appear preoccupied, and avoid conversation.

Physical symptoms may be a major topic of conversation with the treatment staff. Depression causes a preoccupation with one's self and the patient may be come excessively concerned about the body, physical health, and kidney functioning. Generally, sleep disturbances, loss of appetite and weight, vague pains, and dryness of the mouth are common presentations. Transplant patients express excessive concern about urine output, tend to have pelvic pain, or any number of other symptoms that symbolize a concern about the integrity of the kidney.

Changes in social relations, either with friends or with the treatment staff, may be an early sign of depression. In mild depressive states, there can be an actual increase in activities, including bringing gifts to the staff and seeking out conversations. These seem to be a way of buying affection and attention, probably based upon a fear that they are no longer accepted or respected. This may be seen in the newly transplanted patient. The past role as a dialysis patient demanded 10–20 hours per week of attention from the staff. Now with a transplant, the attention received is much, much less and the patient's depression may cause an attempt to reestablish that relationship.

Understanding Depression

Castelnuovo-Tedesco[23] has outlined a useful framework for understanding depressive reactions. First, the depressed patient is portrayed as a disappointed person. Depression is a response to the loss of something, whether it be actual (e.g., a job, social status, a rejected kidney) or whether it is simply a threatened loss or fantasied one (e.g., rejection of the kidney when it is physiologically functioning well). Considering the patient as a disappointed person allows inquiry into the thoughts and actions that have caused disappointment. Does the patient have unfulfilled expectations or, as is often the case, a misinterpretation of the expectations and attitudes of family or staff? What had the patient anticipated posttransplant life to be?

Disappointed persons feel that they have been let down by others or that they have let themselves down. By allowing the patient to express feelings of regret, a clearer understanding of values and expectations that have led to the current emotional status is obtained. Such a reassessment of the situation provides a different perspective, one that allows a lessening of depressed mood. Depression causes a person to suffer passively. They feel immobilized and can see no solution to their problems. For example, the wife of a transplant patient left him shortly after the diagnosis of renal failure. The patient became very depressed in response to the disappointment and abandonment, blaming himself for "driving her off." He quietly endured a brief hemodialysis treatment without complaints or making his depression known. After transplantation he refused to believe that his kidney was functioning well, despite clear evidence to the contrary and maintained a dependent, helpless, sick role while in the hospital. The nursing staff saw his behavior and beliefs as irrational and unreasonable, and attempted to alter them with an inappropriate behavior modification program. Statements about his poor kidney function were responded to with positive comments about his recovery and he was told his physiological data. Excessive requests for care were discouraged with statements about his abilities. The intent was to convince him that he was capable and in good condition. He became even more regressed, childish, clearly depressed, and developed a fever of unknown etiology, all of which prompted a psychiatric consultation. After a detailed history was obtained, he was encouraged to reevaluate the disappointment he felt regarding his abandonment and illness. Some suggestions were made regarding realistic actions that he could take in his marriage and he eventually left the hospital without depression.

Secondly, the depressed person is angry. Such patients receive threat and harm, and because they feel responding is futile, they react emotionally rather than productively to alter the situation. It is important for the staff to explore the hurts and disappointments that have caused the emotion rather than to simply focus on the anger itself. Occasionally we hear the advice "let it all out" or "blow off steam." Encouraging the patient to ventilate anger without understanding its cause does little to relieve the situation and can do much to worsen patients' relationships with others in the environment (e.g., telling off the boss causes one to get fired). Rather, patients should be encouraged to discuss all of the underlying issues, whether real or fantasized, in order to reassess them.

A third generalization about depression is that it involves a sense of guilt. Patients feel unworthy, lack self-esteem, and feel that they have lost the approval of their important friends and family. For transplant patients a major source of this guilt concerns the thoughts and attitudes about the kidney donor. The transplant patient may distort some casual comment that was made to the donor and remember it as a statement that pressured the donor to give up a precious kidney. Guilt causes recipients to doubt their being worthy of the gift. For example, a female transplant recipient became very depressed following her surgery, despite the excellent function of her kidney, because of guilt feelings over her belief that she had deprived her 16-year-old daughter of a mother–daughter relationship while on dialysis. The feelings of guilt and their emotional repercussions surfaced only upon her imminent return to a normal relationship. Such secret thoughts often underlie guilt.

A fourth generalization about depression is a feeling of dependency and helplessness. Depression causes people to lose confidence in their ability to handle day-to-day activities and problems. They remember their dependent posture vis-a-vis hemodialysis and anticipate a similar occurrence with a transplanted kidney. Doubt, uncertainty, and quite often a mistrust are basic characteristics of these individuals. It is helpful at this stage to urge the patient to review past accomplishments and activities that were enjoyed. Gradually, an image of a person who has positive features, who has strengths as well as weaknesses, emerges. The depressed patient's self-image is generally so negative that one's judgment about self and circumstances are distorted.

Techniques of Interaction

As stated previously, it is the intent of this chapter to encourage the participation of the transplant service in psychotherapeutic activities by utilizing their untutored skills of interest, friendliness, and common sense. The reader interested in techniques of interaction in brief supportive psychotherapy is referred to detailed reviews by Castelnuovo-Tedesco,[24] Sifneos,[25] and Wolberg.[26] However, some basic aspects of brief psychotherapy deserve mention in this chapter.

Brief psychotherapy is aimed at the person's current emotional status and tends to be predominately symptom and situation oriented. Attempts at reconstructing or altering the basic personality style are avoided. Realistically, an alteration of the individual's basic personality characteristics is not feasible within the context of brief meetings. Of more importance is the likelihood that such a goal or orientation in the therapy sessions will do little to relieve patient suffering. The patient's basic defenses, whatever they may be, should be supported rather than a change being attempted.

Secondly, a depressed patient needs an active therapist rather than a nondirective approach. They are looking for answers and they need to understand their problems. While they may know the facts of the situation, they seldom have an appreciation of the significance or impact of these events. As stated previously, many of these patients do not even recognize that they are depressed and by pointing out their emotional status they are provided assurance and support.

It is also essential to gain an adequate history of the patient's significant losses and disappointments so that they may be discussed with the patient. Which of their many expectations have not been met? What is the anticipated future with the new transplanted organ?

Patients should be reoriented from their negative attitudes and encouraged to be aware of their strengths and assets. Assistance should be directed to achieving a more balanced and realistic view of themselves by pointing out positive features despite their negative views.

Discussion with depressed patients is more time consuming than with other individuals. They take longer to respond and they may lose track of their train of thought. The staff should recognize these features and avoid becoming bored or even annoyed with the patient's interactive style. Sympathizing and reviewing the topics that have occurred so far will allow the patient to regroup and continue. It is important to remember that depressed patients seek feedback, suggestions, and perspectives. They are looking for more than a listening post.

CONCLUSIONS

In this chapter the activity of the entire transplant service in psychotherapeutic pursuits has been encouraged. The use of group discussions for patients and family, with patient education as a core theme, can serve as a major thrust in the prevention and alleviation of emotional distress. Depression is the most frequent psychological problem encountered in this patient population and it proves to be amenable to brief supportive psychotherapy, a technique capably applied by the transplant service. It should be reiterated that the goal of psychotherapeutic interaction with the transplant patient is to assist in the relief of suffering by attempting to understand the nature of the problem and to suggest appropriate remedial action. Referral to a qualified psychotherapist may be the appropriate solution. However, it is in the interest of good patient care for the entire transplant service to recognize that all of their patient interactions have psychotherapeutic properties. With interest and a modest investment of time, these interactions can reap enormous psychological gains.

REFERENCES

1. MILNE, J. F. Psychosocial aspects of renal transplantation. *Urology* (supplement), 1977, 9, 82–88.
2. ABRAM, H., and BUCHANAN, D. C. The gift of life: a review of the psychological aspects of kidney transplantation. *International Journal of Psychiatry in Medicine*, 1976–77, 7, 153–164.
3. COLLINS, J. L. Multidisciplinary consultation for a renal dialysis-kidney transplantation unit. *Journal of the National Medical Association*, 1974, 66, 277–280.
4. KEMPH, J. P. Renal failure, artificial kidney and kidney transplant. *American Journal of Psychiatry*, 1966, 122, 1270–1274.
5. KEMPH, J. P. Psychotherapy with patients receiving kidney transplant. *American Journal of Psychiatry*, 1967, 124, 623–629.
6. HEALY, K. M. Does preoperative instruction make a difference? *American Journal of Nursing*, 1968, 68, 62–67.
7. LINDEMAN, C. A., and VAN AERMAN, B. Nursing intervention with the presurgical patient: The effect of structured and unstructured preoperative teaching. *Nursing Research*, 1971, 20, 319–332.
8. EGBERT, L. C. Reduction of post operative pain by encouragement and instruction of patients. *New England Journal of Medicine*, 1964, 270, 825–827.
9. NICKERSON, D. Teaching the hospitalized diabetic. *American Journal of Nursing*, 1972, 75, 935–938.
10. PRATT, J. H. The class method of treating consumption in the homes of the poor. *Journal of the American Medical Association*, 1907, 49, 755–759.
11. PATTISON, E. M., RHODES, R. J., and DUDLEY, D. L. Response to group treatment in patients with severe chronic lung disease. *International Journal of Group Psychotherapy*, 1971, 21, 214–225.
12. SHAMBAUGH, P. W., and KANTER, S. S. Spouses under stress: Group meetings with spouses of patients on hemodialysis. *American Journal of Psychiatry*, 1969, 125, 928–936.
13. FORD, C. V. and LONG, K. D. Group psychotherapy of somatizing patients. *Psychotherapy and Psychosomatics*, 1977, 28, 294–304.
14. BUCHANAN, D. C. Group therapy for kidney transplant patients. *International Journal of Psychiatry in Medicine*, 1975, 6, 523–531.
15. HOLLON, T. H. Modified group therapy in the treatment of patients on chronic hemodialysis. *American Journal of Psychotherapy*, 1972, 26, 501–510.
16. HARTINGS, M. F., PAVLOU, M. M., and DAVIS, F. A. Group counseling of M.S. patients in a program of comprehensive care. *Journal of Chronic Diseases*, 1976, 29, 65–73.
17. BROCK, D., LAWSON, R. K., and BENNETT, W. M. Preoperative workshops with patients waiting for kidney transplants.   *Transplant Proceedings*, 1973, 5, 1059–1060.
18. GUSSOW, Z., and TRACY, G. S. The role of self-help clubs in adaptation to chronic illness and disability. *Social Science and Medicine*, 1976, 10, 407–414.
19. BUCHANAN, D. C. Group therapy for chronic physically ill patients. *Psychosomatics*, 1978, 19, 425–431.
20. PENN, I., BUNCH, D., OLENIK, D., and ABOUNA, G. M. Psychiatric experiences with

patients receiving renal and hepatic transplants. In P. Castelnuovo-Tedesco (Ed.), *Psychiatric aspects of organ transplantation*. New York: Grune and Stratton, 1971.
21. ABRAM, H., MOORE, G. L., and WESTERVELT, F. B. Suicidal behavior in chronic dialysis patients. *American Journal of Psychiatry*, 1971, 127, 1199–1204.
22. KEMPH, J. P. Obervations of the effects of kidney transplant on donors and recipients. *Diseases of the Nervous System*, 1970, 31, 323–325.
23. CASTELNUOVO-TEDESCO, P. Brief psychotherapy of depression. In J. O. Cole, A. F. Schatzberg, and S. H. Frazier (Eds.), *Depression: biology, psychodynamics and treatment*. New York: Plenum Press, 1978.
24. CASTELNUOVO-TEDESCO, P. Brief psychotherapy. In D. X. Freedman and J. E. Dyrud (Eds.), *American handbook of psychiatry*. Vol. 5, New York: Basic Books, 1975.
25. SIFNEOS, P. E. *Short-term psychotherapy and emotional crisis*. Cambridge: Harvard University Press, 1972.
26. WOLBERG, L. R. *Short-term psychotherapy*. New York: Grune and Stratton, 1965.

Index

Abandonment, 75, 88, 186, 273
Abram, H. S., 5, 7–8, 33, 34, 43, 46, 49, 50, 59, 77, 100, 104, 106, 109, 110, 115, 146, 175, 197, 217, 221, 224, 271, 276, 277
Acceptance of transplant, 185–193
Acting out, 118, 128, 259
Adaptation (see also Maladaptation), 24, 27, 30, 39, 40, 43, 72
  of children, 80, 85, 177–182
  to hemodialysis, 105, 107, 117–132, 133, 169–175
  long-term, 106, 213
  to transplantation, 195, 196, 204, 207, 210, 216
Affects, see Anger, Anxiety, Depression, etc.
Age, 148, 162, 240
Aggression, 98, 118, 128, 135, 136, 137, 139, 156, 164, 222, 256
  in children, 178, 179, 180, 182
Aging, 21, 220
Ainsworth, M. D. S., 182
Ambivalence, 71, 86, 95, 117, 144, 251
  donors, 186, 229, 233, 234, 235, 239, 240
  family relationship, 84, 237–238, 240
  pretransplant, 74, 238–239, 241
  recipients, 187
  sex roles, 234–237
American Protestant Hospital Association, 61
Ames, S. B., 182
Amputation, 219, 220
Anderson, R. B., 61–70
Anemia, 3, 5, 6, 55
Anger, 40–41, 63, 66, 67, 69, 75, 82, 83, 86, 87, 88, 171, 202, 205, 209, 266, 271, 273
Anorexia, 14
Anovulation, 44
Anthony, S., 182

Antidepressants, 46
Antoniou, L. D., 44, 46
Anxiety, 25, 28, 29, 30, 49, 55, 56, 72, 75, 82, 85, 89, 122–123, 128, 136, 137, 149, 150, 155, 156, 160, 162–165, 170, 175, 177, 180, 181, 196, 197, 199, 203, 211, 214, 215, 220, 223, 224, 256, 261, 269
  recognition of, 271–275
Apathy, 134, 197, 271
Armstrong, S., 247–253
Asterixis, 14
Attention span, 14
Attitude
  to death, 170, 174
  of donors, 238–239, 242–243
  of patient, 22, 51, 171
  of staff, 125–127, 129–130
Attractiveness, 158
Autonomic impairment, 14
Azotemia, 3, 6

Bacterial enzymes, 4, 11
Balck, F., 147–167
Balint, M., 144, 146, 261, 262
Basch, S. H., 93–100, 107, 186, 192, 217, 222, 224, 252
Beard, B. H., 146, 169–175, 197, 217
Beavert, C. S., 146
Beckmann, D., 148, 157, 166
Behavior (see also specific terms, i.e., Aggression, Coping, Suicide, etc.), 22, 28, 30, 36, 37, 38, 41, 119, 134, 143, 247, 272
  change, 13, 85, 90
  modification, 57, 128, 129
Bell Adjustment Inventory, 170, 171
Bennett, W. M., 267, 276
Berkman, A. H., 46, 47
Bernstein, D. M., 91, 186, 193, 240, 245

This Index was prepared by June G. Rosenberg, Senior Assistant Librarian, Medical Research Library of Brooklyn, Downstate Medical Center.